"As advances in medicine help us to live longer, we now face the challenge of how to maintain our vitality, often while also dealing with various chronic conditions. Increasingly, yoga is being recognized as a way to improve and maintain one's mental and physical health when practiced in a safe and appropriate way. In *Relax into Yoga for Seniors*, Kimberly Carson and Carol Krucoff provide the program all seniors need to integrate yoga into their lives and improve their health and well-being."

—**Adam Perlman, MD,** executive director at Duke
Integrative Medicine, and associate vice president at
Duke Health and Wellness

"Kimberly Carson and Carol Krucoff are two of the most trusted, and trustworthy, voices in the field of therapeutic yoga. *Relax into Yoga for Seniors* is a perfect introductory guide not just to yoga, but to a philosophy of embracing the changes that come with age. This book and the practices described will help you find the strength, energy, and ease to engage with life fully."

—**Kelly McGonigal, PhD,** health psychologist at
Stanford University, and author of *Yoga for Pain Relief*

"*Relax into Yoga for Seniors* is a well-researched and thoughtful book that leverages the authors' many years of practice experience as well as their work and close ties with the world of integrative medicine. It provides older adults with a practical, effective compendium of yoga practices that they can readily adopt. Whether they are well or experiencing distressing chronic conditions, *Relax into Yoga for Seniors*' practices can enhance their quality of life."

> —**John W. Graham, PhD**, senior investigator at the University of North Carolina at Chapel Hill's Gillings School of Global Public Health

"*Relax into Yoga for Seniors* brings together Kimberly Carson and Carol Krucoff's experience in teaching their *Integrative Yoga for Seniors Professional Training* at Duke Integrative Medicine. It describes a step-by-step approach to yoga for healthy aging and how to relax into yoga. This is a masterpiece book, which should be an essential resource for seniors, health care professionals, and yoga practitioners, who will find themselves coming back to the text time and time again for deeper study and practice.

> —**Dilip Sarkar, MD, FACS, CAP**, associate professor of surgery (retired) at Eastern Virginia Medical School; fellow at the American Association of Integrative Medicine (AAIM) and American College of Surgeons (ACS); president of the International Association of Yoga Therapists (IAYT); and chairman of board at Life in Yoga Institute

"Carson and Krucoff have skillfully taken the complex, confusing world of yoga and made it practical for anyone, not just seniors. The 'magic' is that in simplifying from their many years of practice with seniors, they have solved how to make yoga safe and effective for the full spectrum of abilities in this diverse population. *Relax into Yoga for Seniors* needs to be embossed onto every prescription pad printed!"

—**Matthew J. Taylor, PT, PhD**, yoga safety expert and past
president of the International Association of Yoga Therapists
www.smartsafeyoga.com

"In this inspiring and accessible book, Kimberly Carson and Carol Krucoff offer you peaceful ways to prioritize your positivity and wellness. Relax and enjoy!"

—**Barbara L. Fredrickson, PhD**, Kenan Distinguished Professor of
psychology and neuroscience at the University of North Carolina
at Chapel Hill, and author of *Positivity* and *Love 2.0*

"Yoga, as a mind-body practice or a way of life, is transformative and leads to improved health, wellness, and connection to self and others. A daily yoga practice is especially important to foster healthy aging. *Relax into Yoga for Seniors* is a wonderful guide to help people start practicing yoga at any age."

—**Lorenzo Cohen, PhD**, professor and director of the Integrative
Medicine Program at The University of Texas MD Anderson Cancer
Center, and coeditor of *Principles and Practice of Yoga in Health Care*

Relax into Yoga *for* Seniors

A Six-Week Program for Strength, Balance, Flexibility, and Pain Relief

KIMBERLY CARSON, MPH, E-RYT
CAROL KRUCOFF, E-RYT

New Harbinger Publications, Inc.

Publisher's Note

This publication is designed to provide accurate and authoritative information in regard to the subject matter covered. It is sold with the understanding that the publisher is not engaged in rendering psychological, financial, legal, or other professional services. If expert assistance or counseling is needed, the services of a competent professional should be sought.

Distributed in Canada by Raincoast Books

Copyright © 2016 by Kimberly Carson and Carol Krucoff
New Harbinger Publications, Inc.
5674 Shattuck Avenue
Oakland, CA 94609
www.newharbinger.com

Cover design by Amy Shoup

Acquired by Jess O'Brien

Edited by Marisa Solís

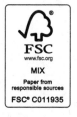
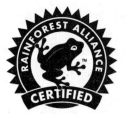

Library of Congress Cataloging-in-Publication Data on file

18   17   16

10   9   8   7   6   5   4   3   2   1   First Printing

"Asana must have the dual qualities of alertness and relaxation."

—*Patanjali's Yoga Sutras*, translated by T. K. V. Desikachar

With great love and respect, we dedicate this work to our elders. Thank you for teaching us about the depth and mystery of aging and the resiliency of spirit.

I Would Rather Make Wine of Life

I have died a thousand times
clinging to life.
Breath stops
and muscles go rigid
trying to freeze frame it,
do it over again,
reshape it,
perfect it,
be better.

I am done wrestling the life out of my experience.
I would rather make wine of life.

Each experience juicy and unique,
ripe, picked, squeezed, savored.
Not about perfection,
for it is the mixture of all these flavors
that makes wine sweet,
an elixir to be shared with friends
as we sit around smiling,
saying "That was a good year."
"Aged well."

—Rebecca Folsom, from *Your Life Is a Masterpiece*

Contents

Foreword

It takes a long time to become young.

—Pablo Picasso

"A seventy-eight-year-old man walks into a yoga class" may sound like the opening line of a joke, but with *Relax into Yoga for Seniors*, Kimberly Carson and Carol Krucoff propel us from contemporary stereotypes of aging onto an extraordinary bridge between modern Western culture and ancient Eastern mind-body-spirit traditions. This novel bridge literally opens a transformative gateway to those of us who continuously redefine "seniors" as "everyone else at least ten years older than me."

For almost a decade, Kimberly Carson and Carol Krucoff have matured a unique approach, teaching Western yoga instructors the adaptation of yoga practice through their "Therapeutic Yoga for Seniors" programs at Duke Integrative Medicine/Duke University Medical Center. Now the authors offer their combined practical skills and vision directly to those of us older folk whose breathing, mobility, strength, flexibility, balance, joy, and overall peace of mind may feel impinged upon by our aging, by pain, or simply by the effort to avoid feeling lost in the midst of an ever-accelerating Western civilization.

Factually, as the authors point out, seniors are the most rapidly growing sector of the Western population. As most of us will come to experience, Western culture spends far more time considering what to do with the elderly—costs of health care, high-tech tools to further extend life, specialized facilities to manage their care—than it spends considering elders as sources of wisdom or lynchpins for family and community. And even in our "eighty is the new fifty" era, neither our culture nor our medical sciences have a ready understanding of what an optimal approach to extended life spans actually entails.

Also factually, the progression of age through senior years brings with it an excruciating Western medical calculus. Just by virtue of age, seniors are more likely to develop infirmities of the body—high blood pressure, heart trouble, stroke and neurologic disorders, arthritis, bone fractures, and kidney and lung disease, just to name a few. And, just by virtue of age, seniors are more likely to both develop complications from their disorders and suffer complications from the pills and surgeries used to treat those disorders.

Spiritually, not surprisingly, Western seniors thus commonly experience aging in daily life as an ineluctable path of progressive debility, powerlessness, and isolation—a lived experience palpably connoting "the end of days." Immersed in such daily experience, this sense of the fading of the flesh is often managed with the mind's most reductionist dark-humor baseball bats, such as "aging is not for wimps," or "aging stinks, but it beats the alternative."

But aging does not have to be this way, and *Relax into Yoga for Seniors* provides a comfortable and accessible guide to transforming our senior years into a very different physical, mental, and spiritual life experience.

Kimberly and Carol reach out to seniors beginning with the most familiar and comfortable crossroad of East and West: the breath. They invite seniors to begin wherever we are in the moment—whether in pain, recovering from a procedure, feeling stiff as a board, or feeling pretty good and wanting to stay that way or better. The authors guide us to approach aging not as an evolving disability but as an enriched and natural time for a new beginning. This deep resource uniquely empowers us to pursue a personal practice of healing and growth.

Perhaps most important, they reach out to us with an antidote to Western aging's social and personal isolation: reconnecting us within; turning the mind to heal the body; turning the body to heal the mind; turning the practice of yoga, centered around the very breaths that we draw, into a process of revitalizing the Spirit. And through revitalizing mind, body, and Spirit, yoga practice promotes a reconnection to the world around us, recovering the world as a place where beauty, joy, and the wisdom of elders not only coexist but actively complement one another.

The authors also recognize another unique dimension of the reality for Western seniors interested in yoga: physical safety. Unlike Eastern seniors, for whom yoga *asanas* (postures) or tai chi forms may be practiced from childhood into life's later stages, Western seniors interested in yoga for the very first time warrant more personalized approaches to beginning a safe, steady, and joyful practice. Kimberly and Carol thus emphasize awareness of the body, including some fundamental knowledge about how the body changes with age relevant to initiating a yoga practice in later stages of life.

These important safety principles are fully contextualized in the vision of the real fruits of relaxing into yoga: gently advancing breathing capacity, strength, mobility, balance, and awareness itself, from wherever we begin today toward a more vital, fluent, connected, and empowered presence in both our inner and outer worlds. This gentle book provides a bridge between East and West, an ancient path adapted particularly to transform "the end of days" into the blossoming of a new stage of life and living in the modern Western world. Why *would* a seventy-eight-year-old man walk into a yoga class…indeed. Read on.

—Mitchell W. Krucoff, MD, FACC, FAHA, FSCAI
Professor, Medicine/Cardiology
Duke University Medical Center/Duke Clinical Research Institute

The Evolution of Therapeutic Yoga for Seniors

Every individual brings a unique constellation of physical, emotional, and spiritual needs and abilities to the yoga practice—a truth that was highlighted as we began teaching yoga in medical settings nearly two decades ago.

A typical class at Duke University's Health and Fitness Center, for example, might include a twenty-year-old soccer player, a seventy-year-old heart attack survivor, a thirty-five-year-old with chronic back pain, a sixty-year-old with advanced cancer, and a forty-five-year-old competitive swimmer. As a hospital-based wellness center, the facility attracted older adults with heart conditions and other ailments who felt safer in this environment than in a typical gym. But it also drew fit underclassmen and professors, plus athletes of all ages. Beginners stood next to experienced practitioners, fit folks alongside deconditioned ones, grandmothers by college students.

Facing this array of diversity was a humbling and deeply educational experience, and creating a yoga class that met the needs of this varied group was ultimately extremely rewarding. It forced us to dig deep into the heart of the teachings and to let go of preconceived and commonly held notions of what a yoga practice entails so that we could open up to the joyful creativity and vast potential inherent in the experience of yoga. It also led us to realize that we were navigating uncharted territory. While yoga is an ancient wisdom tradition, the modern yoga class is a relatively new phenomenon. Back when the yogic practices evolved, there weren't large communities of people ages sixty and up. And ancient yoga teachers didn't have students with artificial joints or implanted defibrillators, or who were taking numerous prescription medications.

This experience led us to search for further training so that we could learn how to best ensure the safety of our more vulnerable students. But we could find no programs that would help us understand the various health problems our more mature students faced and teach us the movement considerations that are essential to making the posture practices both safe and effective. Nor could we find educational opportunities that would help us better understand the existential concerns that often become highlighted later in life.

In 2007, we began our partnership with faculty from the Duke University Health System by launching our first professional training, "Teaching Yoga to Seniors." This weekend workshop was held at Duke Integrative Medicine, which had just opened its doors as a state-of-the-art facility providing patient-centered health care that integrates conventional medicine with evidence-based complementary practices such as mindfulness, acupuncture, massage, and yoga. We hoped other yoga teachers would be interested in this three-day workshop featuring talks by Duke medical experts along with interactive sessions on how to adapt the yogic practices to comply with any contraindications and concerns raised by our Duke colleagues. The workshop quickly filled and was extremely successful—but clearly it was too short.

The following year we experimented with a five-day program, then in 2009 we settled on an eight-day version called "Therapeutic Yoga for Seniors" that featured presentations from internationally recognized physicians, physical therapists, and health psychologists geared to providing yoga teachers with the essential fundamentals to work safely and effectively with older adults.

In addition to what we refer to as the "Master Program" at Duke, we also offer some abridged programs held at the Kripalu Center for Yoga and Health, in Massachusetts, as well as at several other locations. We launched a website, Yoga4Seniors.com, with a mission to advance the art and science of adapting the yoga practice to older bodies, minds, and spirits. More than seven hundred yoga teachers from around the world have attended our trainings, and it is our experience that—as pioneers charting this new territory—we are all teaching each other as well as teaching our students.

Relax into Yoga for Seniors is a collaborative effort, and we each bring special talents to the program we have built. We have traveled very different paths to arrive at this place together. Here are our stories.

Kimberly's Story

When I was a small girl, my grandmother was the adult with whom I felt best. She was a most generous and funny soul, and I always felt loved and fully seen by her sweet gaze. Her commitment to and love for me was unwavering, and this experience instilled in me a deep wish to support our elders.

In my early twenties I stumbled into a 6:00 a.m. yoga class held at the only wellness center in town. Trying to relate to so many parts of myself in new and engaging ways was beyond intriguing. It wasn't long before I experienced what might be called an awakening, or moment of clarity, in which a fundamental but previously unrecognized aspect of myself—a steady and ever-present observer, right at my core—made itself known to me. It was almost as if the yoga practice had woken me up to a powerful part of myself that I had always taken for granted and simply overlooked. From that point on, I immersed myself in the teachings and practices of the yoga tradition, which have helped me cultivate emotional intelligence and relate differently to my inner processes.

While working toward my master's degree in public health, I had a surprising and profound deepening into the yoga tradition through the meeting of my future husband, Jim Carson. Before returning to graduate school in his forties, Jim had lived for twenty-two years as a swami (a monk in the yoga tradition) and had taught the philosophy and practices of yoga around the world. As we fell in love and began weaving our lives together, our home became an ongoing immersion in the teachings and practices of yoga.

After earning my master's, I taught yoga classes and mindfulness-based stress reduction at the Duke Health and Fitness Center for more than a decade. Through teaching these classes of mostly older adults, my students became some of my greatest teachers. They helped me better understand their strengths and limitations, as well as what aspects of the yoga practice were most valuable to them. Rather than pursuing accelerated levels of fitness or achieving contortionist postures, functional health was very important: students wanted to enjoy their families, participate in their communities, and find ease in their bodies. In service of optimal function, students reported that the ability to relax, to be steady in the moment, and to deepen their awareness of themselves were also compelling aspects of the practice.

After completing his doctorate in clinical health psychology from the University of North Carolina–Chapel Hill, Jim completed his postdoctoral fellowship in psychiatry and behavioral sciences at Duke, where we collaborated on research evaluating the effects of loving-kindness meditation on chronic low-back pain. While we were there, we became involved with an extraordinary group of clinicians who embarked on a path that explored how to scientifically study the efficacy of the yoga and mindfulness practices, especially for people struggling with medical challenges.

Much of this research is based on the premise that healing can take many forms: more ease, more acceptance, more joy, more forgiveness. It also may result in better physical function and emotional resiliency, even in the face of challenging circumstances. Our research trials have demonstrated that the gentle movements, conscious relaxation, and cultivation of present-moment awareness can reduce the difficult symptoms of pain, fatigue, and emotional distress that occur with many medical conditions.

This experience has reinforced for me not only the utility of these practices for the alleviation of suffering but also the importance of remembering that often the simplest awareness tools can be the most profound. Twenty years of teaching people to pause, notice, and breathe has shown me over and over again that these gestures are often the most powerful yoga practices of all. The power of these gestures has also been invaluable in raising our boy/girl twins. Often what they need most from us as parents is our commitment to pause, breathe, and notice the beauty and vision that they bring to the world. Ultimately, yoga illuminates our relationships—relationship to self, relationships to others—and provides us the ability to clearly see the potential and fullness of life.

Carol's Story

Working at the *Washington Post* in the 1970s and 1980s was a journalist's dream. I was in my twenties and spent long hours in the newsroom, where our legendary editor, Ben Bradlee, encouraged a competitive atmosphere that he called "creative tension." While I adored my job, the stress of vying for plum assignments and hammering out stories on deadline led me to develop chronic neck pain. Searching for relief, I turned to yoga.

My weekly yoga class became an oasis of calm in my life, and I loved the exploration of new positions—like handstand—that literally turned my world upside down. Over time I began to realize that yoga offered much more than stress relief and flexibility. Yoga is a journey of self-discovery, and I found that the lessons I learned tackling challenging postures on the yoga mat helped me navigate more skillfully through challenging situations at work and at home.

In 1988 my family and I moved from Washington, D.C., to Chapel Hill, North Carolina, where my husband, Mitchell Krucoff, joined the cardiology faculty of Duke University Medical Center. One of the first things I did was find a yoga class. By then I had two small children and worked as a freelance writer. When my kids took up karate, I studied martial arts with them—earning my black belt at age forty-two—all the while continuing to take a weekly yoga class.

In 1998 I enrolled in a two-year yoga teacher-training program because I wanted to deepen my yoga practice. To earn our certificates, we were required to complete twelve weeks of community service, and I volunteered teaching yoga in a gerontology rehabilitation program at the Durham Veterans Administration Medical Center. Although I'd been teaching yoga for a year by that time, I found myself very uneasy facing a roomful of elderly male veterans—and a few women—with a wide array of health issues.

Uncertain about what would be appropriate to teach them, I observed their calisthenics class and found that many of their floor exercises were similar to yoga poses. I started there, teaching these familiar positions while adding the breath and the yogic approach of balancing effort with surrender. The group loved the class, and I found it an incredibly rewarding experience. I became known as "The Yoga Lady," and instead of stopping after twelve weeks I continued volunteering for five years.

When Duke Integrative Medicine opened its doors in 2006, I began teaching yoga classes and offering individual yoga sessions in this extraordinary facility. The administrators were open to proposals for programs utilizing this unique environment, and Kimberly and I approached them with our idea of creating a professional training for yoga teachers. In the fall of 2007, we launched "Therapeutic Yoga for Seniors."

As my body has changed with age, I have come to value the well-known saying "We teach what we need to learn." Several health crises have given me a personal understanding of yoga's healing power. Drinking too much water during a marathon in Jamaica in 2003 landed me in a four-day coma from low blood sodium (hyponatremia) and gave me a new appreciation for the deeper practices of yoga. Waking up in Duke's neurointensive care unit with no idea how I'd gotten there was a surreal experience. While I couldn't do any yoga postures, I could do breathing practices, meditation, and relaxation, which I found profoundly healing. In 2008, I had open-heart surgery to replace a congenitally abnormal heart valve. Again, my yoga practice was essential in recovering completely to full and vibrant health.

One of yoga's greatest teachings is that everything changes—except the undying spirit—and throughout my forty years of yoga practice I have been learning to embrace this change. This is not always easy, especially when the change involves illness and loss. Yoga has given me the tools to face whatever arises with equanimity, to be grateful for the gift of breath, and to cherish each day. Distilled to its essence, yoga is love.

Our Integrative Approach

While we have traveled different paths on our journey toward our Relax into Yoga approach, we share a common understanding and respect for medical science alongside our deep personal practice of yoga. This has shaped our approach as an integrative program, in line with the emerging arena of *integrative medicine*. Sometimes confused with "alternative medicine"—which refers to approaches used *instead of* Western medical care—"integrative medicine" *combines* mainstream Western medical therapies with complementary therapies for which there is high-quality evidence of safety and effectiveness. It is also a patient-centered approach to care that considers all factors that influence health and wellness—including the physical body, thoughts and emotions, spirituality, nutrition, relationships, and lifestyle.

Similarly, yoga is based on the recognition that all aspects of our being are interconnected, as well as the understanding that the experiences of our bodies, our minds, and our hearts are not separate. In many ways, yoga is ideally suited for those chapters of life when we face issues of aging, illness, and mortality. A central tenet of the practice is this understanding: *I am not the physical form I experience today. I am not my thoughts. I am not my feelings. These come and go. I am the awareness that doesn't change.*

Impermanence is a reality of life, and it is an inherent part of the human journey to grow older. Despite misconceptions that yoga is about perfecting a difficult posture or attaining a certain temporary state of profound calm, the practice is more about developing the relationship with all parts of yourself—including the simplest most essential *you*: presence itself. When the practice begins to cultivate our ability to *simply be*, pain, grief, and loss can be welcomed with a deeper sense of acceptance and equanimity. In turn, this acceptance and equanimity invite us to relax into life.

PART 1

Yoga for Healthy Aging

"For the unlearned, old age is winter; for the learned, it is the season of the harvest."

—Hasidic saying

INTRODUCTION

If You Can Breathe, You Can Relax into Yoga

"I'd love to try yoga, but…"

In almost two decades of teaching yoga in medical settings, we've heard this wistful phrase from countless people who have mistakenly assumed that yoga isn't for them.

"I'm not flexible enough," they shrug sadly. Or they concede, "I can't sit on the floor," or "I'm too old, too heavy, too stiff."

We're quick to assure them that yoga is *not* just for twentysomethings in spandex. Despite the common misconception that you must be able to twist yourself into a pretzel or stand on your head, there's only one thing you need to do to practice yoga and reap its many benefits. You don't have to touch your toes, sit cross-legged, or even get out of bed.

The only thing you need to be able to do to practice yoga is breathe.

And the potential rewards are vast. This ancient discipline has long been recognized as a path to inner peace and as an excellent way to boost strength, balance, and flexibility. Modern research indicates that yoga offers a host of physiological and psychological benefits, including reducing heart rate and blood pressure, relieving anxiety and depression, and easing back pain.[1] While yoga research is in its infancy, numerous studies are examining its therapeutic effects on a broad array of ailments, including heart failure, arthritis, chronic pain, cancer, and Parkinson's disease.[2] Evidence suggests that yoga not only improves health-related quality of life but also enhances walking and balance, muscle strength, cardiovascular health, and sleep,[3] and it may even improve lung function.[4]

> **Yoga is a comprehensive system for transformation that offers freedom from suffering.**

But not all yoga classes are alike, and it's unfortunately common to find people who say that the supposedly healing practice of yoga caused them pain. As teachers specializing in yoga for potentially vulnerable populations, we often hear stories about people having a negative experience in a yoga class—frequently because the class was too difficult for the participant or taught by an inexperienced or poorly trained instructor. Yoga's booming popularity has resulted in a broad array of offerings, including hybrids such as yoga on an exercise ball, as well as classes taught by instructors whose training consists of a weekend yoga workshop. Even yoga instructors who are adequately trained to teach able, fit students typically have a limited understanding of the important safety considerations that Western medicine recognizes as vital when working with "mature" bodies and people with health issues.

Having the extraordinary opportunity to teach yoga at one of the country's leading academic medical centers has helped us recognize the critical need to integrate evidence-based guidelines from modern medical science with the profound wisdom of the ancient yogic tradition. During the past decade we have worked with top medical experts in varied fields—including pain management, cardiology, physical therapy, oncology, pulmonary rehabilitation, exercise physiology, and geriatrics—to develop a safe and effective yoga practice for older adults and people with medical conditions.

We call our approach "Relax into Yoga" because our work with people at midlife and beyond has highlighted the essential need to develop awareness, ease, and a compassionate relationship with the body. In a culture committed to doing, striving, and pushing, Relax into Yoga cultivates the critical counterbalance of undoing, of slowing down, of savoring the moment and knowing more fully what life is presenting *right now*.

Too often, people are hypercritical of themselves or even at war with their own bodies—saying they "hate" parts of themselves that carry excess weight, feel a little creaky, or experience pain. They might struggle and complain about a "bad" knee or "bum" back, an attitude that can create excess tension and exacerbate pain.

We emphasize learning to treat yourself with kindness, let go of judgment, and to love yourself as you are. Slowing down and paying attention—not only to the physical body but also to emotional and mental reactions—helps calm the nervous system while cultivating strength and flexibility. Making peace with your body—even those places that are "challenged"—can relieve the suffering caused by resistance to the experience you are already having. And rather than working toward complex postures that might be eye-catching on a magazine cover, we focus on poses designed to help people function better in daily life activities, such as walking along a narrow street, carrying groceries, and getting into and out of a car.

We've had the privilege of teaching yoga to countless older adults—ranging from competitive athletes to couch potatoes—as well as those facing serious illness such as cancer, heart failure, and lung disease. Many of our students tell us that yoga has made a profound difference in their health, relieving pain, boosting mood, and enhancing sleep. We hear numerous examples of how yoga has improved their quality of life, from being able to get down on the floor to play with grandchildren, to restoring the ability to play tennis or golf, to being better able to

> **Our Relax into Yoga program cultivates the critical counterbalance of undoing, of slowing down, of savoring the moment and knowing more fully what life is presenting *right now*.**

manage stressful events. And we've seen some dramatic effects of the practice, including students who've been able to cut back or eliminate medications, rely less on the use of a cane, and learn to breathe—rather than scream—through a pain crisis.

While we originally targeted our Relax into Yoga classes for seniors, we've found that many younger people are also drawn to this approach to practice.

Typically these are students facing health issues—such as PTSD, obesity, and chronic pain—who are worried about getting injured or feeling uncomfortable in a "regular" yoga class. It has become clear that our mindful, gentle approach—with a specific focus on safety and effectiveness—can appeal to anyone of any age.

In our wired, worried society, where more than one in five American adults takes at least one mental heath medication,[5] learning to take an easy breath, to quiet your body and mind, and to connect with your innermost self can be a lifesaving skill. We invite you to relax into yoga—a breath-by-breath, step-by-step path to wholeness.

Tailored for Older Adults

We are in the midst of one of the greatest sociological shifts in history: global aging. Sometimes called the "Silver Tsunami" or the "Age Wave," this phenomenon of increased longevity among unprecedented numbers of people promises to dramatically transform our world. Seniors ages sixty-five and older comprise the fastest-growing sector of the U.S. population.[6] This group is expected to more than double (from 8 percent of Americans to 20 percent) to more than eighty million by the year 2050.[7] And there will be a huge jump in the "oldest old"—nearly 5 percent of Americans will be eighty-five and older in 2050, compared to just over 1 percent in 1994.[8, 9]

Like many people looking to boost their health, fitness, and peace of mind, older adults are increasingly drawn to yoga. Yoga is one of the most commonly used complementary health approaches in the nation, with participation nearly doubling from 5.1 percent of adults in 2002 to 9.5 percent in 2012.[10] And a growing number of physicians are encouraging their patients to try yoga to relieve problems such as back pain, high blood pressure, and irritable bowel syndrome. Yet finding a yoga class that is appropriate for baby boomers and beyond can be a challenge.

Most yoga books and studios rely on postures geared to younger individuals—some of which pose potentially serious risks for mature bodies. For example, the popular Sun Salutation sequence includes straight-legged forward bends, a movement that can strain the back and that the National Osteoporosis Foundation advises people with compromised bone to avoid, as it increases the risk of vertebral fracture.[11] People with osteoarthritis in their knees and/or hips often experience pain in postures that place body weight on an affected joint, such as deep squats or sitting cross-legged. And popular "hot yoga" studios that heat the room to temperatures as high as 104 degrees Fahrenheit may be problematic for people with heart disease, particularly those taking medications that can exaggerate the body's response to heat.[12]

Today's seniors are a very diverse group, including healthy and fit individuals able to run marathons, compete in masters athletic events, and even stand on their heads. However, much more common are those who fit the profile of an average seventy-five-year-old in America: someone who has three chronic conditions and uses five prescription drugs.[13] Many of the medications taken for common conditions such as high blood pressure, pain, and depression can increase the risk of falling.[14] Among people over sixty-five, falls are the number one cause of fractures, hospital admissions for trauma, loss of independence, and injury deaths.[15] That's why it's essential to make sure your yoga practice is safe, appropriate, and effective. This includes beginners as well as experienced practitioners who want to adapt their practice to their changing bodies, hearts, and minds.

Along with a growing appreciation of yoga's therapeutic benefits has come an increased recognition that, like any physical activity, yoga can cause injury. Triggered in part by a controversial 2012 *New York Times Magazine* cover story, "How Yoga Can Wreck Your Body," is a burgeoning awareness that the supposedly healing practice of yoga may also cause harm.[16] And, somewhat paradoxically, the very people who may have the most to gain from yoga—older adults and people with health challenges—may also have the most to lose.

> **Yoga offers a host of physiological and psychological benefits, including reducing heart rate and blood pressure, relieving anxiety and depression, and easing back pain.**

Sixty Is the New Forty

When we first started teaching yoga at Duke University and the Durham VA Medical Center in the late 1990s, the idea that yoga was not just for young-sters who wanted to stand on their heads but might actually benefit people fifty and up, as well as those with serious illness, was brand new. This budding inter-est in yoga's healing potential arose, in part, from a groundbreaking study pub-lished in 1990 in one of medicine's top journals, the *Lancet*, suggesting that a yogic lifestyle may stop, slow, or even reverse the progression of heart disease.[17]

This was also a time when medical advances were triggering the new "lon-gevity boom" by helping people recover from ailments that might have killed them just a generation ago. The development of clot-busting drugs, such as tPA, gave physicians a lifesaving tool to combat heart attack and stroke. Today, tens of thousands of Americans survive these events each year and go on to live active, full lives.[18] Advances in oncology have made cancer—once a death sentence—now increasingly survivable, with more than 14 million Americans, most of whom are seniors, having experienced the cancer journey.[19] Many people who have faced such serious health issues describe the experience as a turning point in their lives, prompting them to embrace healthy physical and emotional changes such as exercising and eating well. As a result, they become stronger and more resilient than ever before.

In fact, thanks largely to progress in medicine, *the human life span has almost doubled in the last century.* As recently as 1900, the average life expectancy in the United States was 47.[20] In 2012, that number jumped to an all-time high of 78.8 years: 81.2 for females and 76.4 for males.[21] And in some other countries people live even longer: 87 years for women in Japan and 81.2 years for men in Iceland.[22] Throughout the world, more people are living to more advanced ages than ever before—and with a very broad range of functional capacities and needs.

The popular saying "sixty is the new forty" reflects this reality. In our grand-parents' day, life expectancy was about sixty years.[23] But today, someone cele-brating a sixtieth birthday can expect to live two decades or more, with the potential for making this chapter of life truly the golden years. And as a holistic discipline that touches body, mind, and spirit, yoga can be a profound and transformative practice during this precious time.

Relax into Yoga Basics

Our competitive culture promotes a crazy-busy mentality in which we're taught to give 110 percent, push ourselves to achieve, and always be "in it to win it." Many people—including athletes and soldiers—are even encouraged to "sacrifice their bodies" by training themselves to ignore sensations of discomfort and pain.

Yoga offers powerful tools to help offset this disconnected, forceful, frenetic mind-set by inviting us to pause, listen deeply, and be present for whatever is arising—physically, mentally, and spiritually—in each moment. We are reminded to be grateful for the gift of breath and to connect with our deepest, truest selves.

Yet for many people, shifting gears away from the Western striving and pushing mind-set is often extremely challenging. Lifetime habits of body and mind can make it difficult to ease up, relax, and embrace the yogic attitude of finding an appropriate balance between effort and surrender. Most of us are very good at *doing* but struggle with the very thing we need most: *undoing*.

That's why it's essential to recognize that yoga involves not just *what* you do but also *how* you do it. So if you're showing off for spectators while you perform postures (or watching TV or mentally checking items off your to-do list) the experience is likely to be quite different than if you were practicing these same poses mindfully, with a nonjudgmental attitude of self-discovery, as you tune in to the various dimensions of your inner experience (for example, sensations, thoughts, feelings, energy). Our Relax into Yoga program is designed to help you cultivate a new and/or deeper awareness through yoga postures, breathing, meditation, and principles.

Awareness

Despite the common misconception that yoga is primarily a form of exercise, this ancient discipline is actually a practice of *awareness* designed to quiet your mind and help you connect with your innermost self. Much more than a workout, yoga is a powerful form of mind-body medicine that approaches health in a holistic manner, honoring the interplay of our physical, emotional, and spiritual well-being. At its heart, yoga is a comprehensive system for transformation and freedom from suffering.

Awareness is a central component of yoga and is integral to all aspects of the practice:

Postures. The most well-known part of the yogic toolbox, postures can help strengthen muscles, enhance flexibility, relieve pain, boost balance, and increase your ability to function. The Sanskrit word for posture is *asana*, which means "seat." The practice is designed to cultivate the awareness necessary to finding a "comfortable seat" in each pose.

> **Yoga is a powerful form of mind-body medicine that approaches health in a holistic manner.**

Breathing. The yogic term for "breathing practice" is *pranayama*, which means extension and control of *prana*, the Sanskrit term for "breath," "vital energy," and "life force." Breathing is the only physiologic function controlled by two different sets of nerves and muscles: voluntary and involuntary. You don't have to think about breathing; fortunately, your body will breathe automatically. But when you bring awareness to your breathing, it provides a unique doorway into your central nervous system—the control center that revs you up to fight or flee when you perceive danger, and calms you down when the emergency is over. As the link between the conscious and unconscious mind, breathing practice can help change your physiology and emotional state. For example, slowing the breath and making the exhalation longer than the inhalation can help lower the heart rate and invite the relaxation response. Awareness of our breath is an essential tool in helping us recognize and navigate what is happening in our body, heart, and mind.

Meditation. The process of focusing attention and quieting mental chatter, meditation helps harness the mind-body connection and can transform mental and physical agitation into peacefulness. Although some people become convinced of the idea that meditation requires *emptying* the mind, it actually involves *steadying* the mind with an object of focus—such as the breath, a sound, a prayer, a candle flame, or virtually anything. Typically, the object of meditation is something positive, appealing, and healing, because whatever happens in the mind affects the entire system. Awareness is at the heart of meditation.

Principles. In the West, the yogic guidelines for ethical and moral conduct are probably the least well-known of yoga's tools. Part of the Eightfold Path designed to lead to enlightenment that is outlined in *The Yoga Sutras of Patanjali*, the classic text on yoga, these ten basic guidelines are designed to improve our relationships—with others and with ourselves—which can have a profound impact on our well-being. They are grouped into guidelines for social relationships called *yamas* (nonviolence, truthfulness, non-stealing, sexual continence, and non-hoarding) and for personal conduct called *niyamas* (cleanliness, contentment, discipline, self-study, and surrender to something greater than ourselves). We are encouraged to let our posture practice be informed by these attitudes, for example, avoiding the physical violence of forcing our bodies into a painful position or the emotional violence of abusive self-talk. Yoga's healing power is enhanced when we take these attitudes from our practice into our lives.

> **We emphasize learning to treat yourself with kindness, let go of judgment, and to love yourself as you are.**

The Carson-Krucoff Principles of Practice

In the ancient teachings of yoga, love is considered a central defining virtue of the human experience. To reflect this, we have created specific principles to cultivate a loving approach to every aspect of your practice. This includes how you move into and out of the postures, the quality of your relationship to thoughts and feelings, and your receptivity to energies, sensations, and spirit.

These principles were published in a journal article we wrote with several Duke colleagues that outlines essential considerations involved in teaching yoga to seniors.[24] We have adapted them here to be relevant to students of any age or ability level who are interested in our heart-centered mindful approach to the full dimension of the yoga experience—physical, mental, emotional, and spiritual. (We've also written a teacher's guide that further expands on the Carson-Krucoff principles for those interested in teaching yoga to older adults. Visit http://www.newharbinger.com/33643 to download it.)

1. "First, Do No Harm"

This aligns with the yogic principle of *ahimsa*, or "nonviolence." It applies to more than just physical violence, as it also relates to emotional harm from unkind words or behaviors. If you've ever complained about a "bad" knee or called a part of your body "ugly," this is a kind of violence against yourself. Learning to love yourself, even those parts that are challenged or less than ideal, is central to yoga practice. Avoid violence in your movements as well as in your thoughts, words, and deeds.

2. Create a Safe Environment

Cultivate this attitude of non-harming by not comparing yourself with anyone else, treating yourself kindly, and not forcing your body into painful positions. Avoid being competitive or judgmental.

3. Encourage Yogic Balance

A yoga pose should be "stable and comfortable," according to *The Yoga Sutras of Patanjali*.[25] Challenge yourself in each pose, but avoid strain. Don't be lazy, but don't be pushy, either. Find the middle ground between effort and surrender.

4. Meet Yourself Where You Are

Rather than struggling to perform something you think you *should* be able to do, start where you are and build from there. If an entire pose is too challenging, try just one piece—for example, an arm or leg movement. Even just visualizing yourself making a movement has value.

5. Emphasize Feeling over Form

Let go of ideas of how a pose should look. Focus instead on how a pose feels. Learn to discriminate between *discomfort*, which may be an inherent part of the growth process, and *pain*, which, in general, is to be avoided. *Note:* If you have chronic pain—meaning that you continually live with some amount of pain—it's important not to let pain keep you from moving, because inactivity is likely to exacerbate your pain. But be sure you are doing appropriate postures and breathing practices, and avoid movements that *increase* your level of pain (see "Chronic Pain," page 42).

6. Honor the Inner Teacher

Yoga recognizes that everyone carries a deep, inner wisdom. Learn to listen to this true teacher within, and remember that you are the authority on how you feel. While it can be wise to seek guidance from experts, consider them partners rather than bosses. Recognize that a good yoga teacher is not a drill sergeant but a guide, helping you explore what works best for you.

7. Encourage Gratitude and Joy

Create a mind-set that celebrates what you *can* do. Rather than fixate on what's wrong, consider viewing the situation through the lens of what's right. Cultivate an awareness of your blessings. Approach your prac-

> In the ancient teachings of yoga, love is considered a central defining virtue of the human experience.

13

tice in a manner similar to a child released onto the playground for recess. Have fun moving your body, and enjoy your breath.

8. Emphasize Fluidity

The ancient Chinese text, the Tao Te Ching, teaches that "whoever is soft and yielding is a disciple of life."[26] This is particularly important as the body loses resiliency with age. Avoid jerky, ballistic movements and rigid holdings. Instead, cultivate a fluid quality of movement.

9. Use Skillful Language

Our choice of words holds great power in helping us learn not just *what* to do but also *how* to do it. We encourage you to use skillful language in your self-talk, so your inner dialogue is kind and compassionate as you move toward your own seat of stability and comfort. *Invite* and *encourage* yourself into the practice, rather than *direct* and *demand,* to better facilitate your own personal journey within.

10. The Practice Is About *You*, Not About the Pose

It's not uncommon to come to yoga looking for relief from a troublesome problem such as an achy back, heart disease, or arthritis pain. While yoga may help heal these issues, our approach doesn't focus on the symptom or ailment itself but on the person who is experiencing it. This means that an appropriate yoga practice for one person with back pain may be quite different from the appropriate practice for someone else with a similar problem. Remember that yoga is designed to help you quiet your mind and connect with your true self. Easing physical and emotional distress may be essential to helping you find this union, but it is the experience of union itself that is at the heart of the practice. Ultimately, yoga invites us to take refuge in the simplicity of being, the beauty of presence itself.

How to Use This Book

Relax into Yoga for Seniors is divided into two parts:

Part 1: Yoga for Healthy Aging. Here you'll find important information about yoga and health. The preface describes how we came to create our Relax into Yoga approach through our own need to make the practice safe and effective for our more vulnerable students. The introduction provides an overview of relevant societal shifts and medical advances, and outlines the basic principles of our approach. Chapter 1 offers detailed information on how our bodies change with age. Just as we notice the effects of aging on the outside—graying hair and wrinkled skin, for example—we also experience inner changes that we don't see but may feel as stiffness, loss of resilience, or pain. We explore how physical activity

> Yoga involves not just *what* you do, but also *how* you do it.

is the key to successful aging. Chapter 2 discusses age-related disorders, with specific recommendations for movement considerations essential to people living with these conditions. Feel free to skip around in this chapter and focus on those conditions most relevant to your life. Chapter 3 presents specifics of healthy body mechanics to prevent or relieve common problems such as back and joint pain.

Part 2: Relax into Yoga Practices. These nine chapters will take you on a step-by-step journey to developing your own safe and effective yoga practice. Chapter 4 offers specific, practical guidelines, including how to set up your space and prepare your body and your mind. Chapters 5 through 10 present our six-week program. Each week offers a series of postures plus awareness cues to connect more deeply with your inner experience (thoughts, emotions, breath, sensations, energy) and cultivate a sense of ease. In addition, each week centers around a special focus—including flexibility, back strength, core strength, and balance. Chapter 11 offers additional practices; some are designed to enhance vigor and others to promote relaxation. And chapter 12 provides support for continuing your yoga journey, helping you create your own, personalized practice to suit your goals, interests, and time.

In addition, we have created audio recordings that will guide you through the breathing, postures, and meditations. They are available for free download from our publisher's website at http://www.newharbinger.com/33643. We encourage you to take advantage of this unique resource, since it can be very helpful to be talked through the poses step-by-step once you have reviewed the illustrations and descriptions. This can give you a more fluid practice, as it can be difficult to refer to the book while practicing. (For instructions on how to access the audio recordings, see "How to Get the Accessories for Your Book," on page 229.)

Please read part 1, "Yoga for Healthy Aging," all the way through. In part 2, "Relax into Yoga Practices," spend a week with each chapter. Give yourself time to experience the postures and build the skills presented, such as balance, back strength, and flexibility. Avoid rushing. Make a commitment to give yourself the full six weeks to fully experience our Relax into Yoga program, and then feel free to establish your own program as you become confident in the practice.

May your yoga practice bring you closer and closer to a rich and intimate relationship with yourself and your precious life. Enjoy!

A note for yoga teachers: You may be reading this book as a yoga instructor interested in teaching yoga to older adults but unfamiliar with how to begin adjusting your instruction to safely and effectively work with this population. We've written a guide that will help you do just that: Adapt your teaching for senior students. Visit http://www.newharbinger.com/33643 to access and download our complimentary guide. For instructions on how to do this, see "How to Get the Accessories for Your Book," on page 229.

CHAPTER 1

Yoga for Every Body

Life's one constant is change, and our bodies are a prime example of this continuous flux. Our physical form changes dramatically during our life span: from infancy through childhood, adolescence, and into adulthood; as we grow and mature, gain and lose weight, try on different hairstyles and fashions, experience illness and injury, and—hopefully—return to health. Our bodies also change subtly from day to day (and sometimes moment to moment) depending on many variables, including what we eat, how we sleep, and if we're under stress.

Ideally, yoga practice helps us assess where we are in this changing landscape by bringing awareness to the mind-body connection that allows us to recognize what is true about our physical, mental, and emotional state in any given moment. On the deepest level, yoga also helps unite us with the one unchanging aspect of our experience, which is often referred to as spirit.

Acknowledging the reality of impermanence—the recognition that constant change is a fact of human existence—is a central teaching of the yogic tradition. Honoring this truth, that everything changes, leads to the understanding that becoming attached to something—even the need to practice a yoga posture in a specific way—can lead to suffering. This is a central reason why our Relax into Yoga posture practice includes a continuum of choices for each pose, so you can adjust the posture to meet you where you are

> The only thing you need to be able to do to practice yoga is breathe.

in each practice session—as your body changes day to day and year to year. Yoga also encourages us to cultivate equanimity in the face of changing circumstances, a practice that builds flexibility not only of the joints and muscles but of attitude and outlook.

Movement as Anti-aging Medicine

In general, as people grow older, the heart and blood vessels become stiffer, systems become slower to react and recover, bones weaken, and muscle mass declines. But while aging is inevitable, infirmity is not. One of the best ways to maintain vitality and slow down age-related decline is to keep moving.

But unfortunately, a common reaction to many of life's changes—including getting older—is to stop moving. Typically, this creates a vicious cycle: inactivity leads to deconditioning, which makes movement painful, so you move even less, which makes you stiffer and more deconditioned (and often heavier), which makes movement hurt worse (see figure 1.1). In fact, much of the pain and disability attributed to aging—and to age-related ailments like arthritis—is often actually a result of disuse.

Staying active is one of the best ways to achieve optimum physical and mental health,[27] and yoga's emphasis on adapting the practice to your unique needs in this moment makes it an ideal form of movement for older adults and people with health challenges. It's our belief and experience that *every body, regardless of age or physical limitations, can practice yoga and gain significant benefits.* Aches, pains, and other health problems are not reasons to avoid yoga. On the contrary, the reality that yoga may help relieve, prevent, and sometimes even eliminate many discomforts can be a strong motivator for doing a regular, appropriate yoga practice. And it's never too late to start. Particularly for those in midlife and beyond, the movement, mindfulness, and breath awareness central to yoga practice are powerful tools to boost health, enhance well-being, and age well.

Vicious Cycle of Inactivity

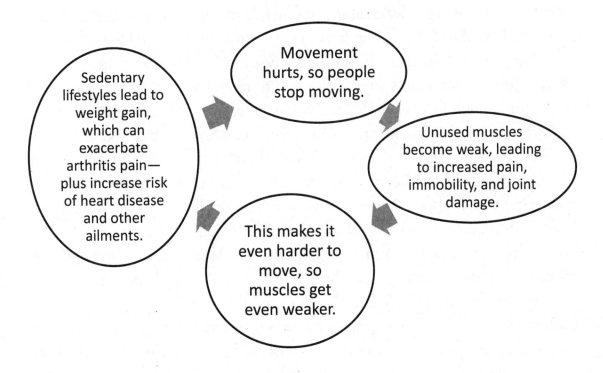

Figure 1.1 Vicious cycle of inactivity

"If exercise could be packed into a pill, it would be the single most widely prescribed and beneficial medicine in the nation," summed up the late gerontologist and Pulitzer Prize–winning author Dr. Robert Butler, who was the first director of the National Institute on Aging.[28] This exercise is particularly important with age. "How we live," Butler wrote in his guide to aging well, *The Longevity Prescription*, "determines a great deal about the pace at which we age."[29]

Movement habits can have a strong effect on the quality of life for people in midlife and beyond. Where and how older adults spend their final years—either vital and living independently or frail in a nursing home—may be greatly influenced by their physical activity habits throughout their lifetime and in their later years. "Current evidence clearly indicates that participation in a regular exercise program is an effective way to reduce and/or prevent a number of the functional declines associated with aging," according to the American College of Sports Medicine's statement on exercise and the older adult.[30]

The benefits of regular, moderate physical activity include everything from boosting health of the heart, lungs, muscles, and bones to managing stress, improving mood, and preventing or delaying many diseases and disabilities.[31] Brain health may also get a boost from being active, as emerging research suggests exercise may play a role in reducing risk for Alzheimer's disease and age-related cognitive decline.[32] "The health improvements with physical activity are often greater than many drugs," notes the UK's Academy of Medical Royal Colleges in a 2015 report urging physicians to promote the "miracle cure" of exercise. "The effect is seen with small amounts of physical activity: 30 minutes, 5 times a week."[33]

In fact, for older adults, increases in physical activity may be as important as quitting smoking for reducing the risk of death.[34] But the sad reality is that less than half (49 percent) of all adults meet the public health recommendations for aerobic exercise, and just one in five (20 percent) gets the recommended amount of aerobic and muscle-strengthening activity.[35] And among adults sixty-five and older, just 12 percent of men and 9 percent of women get the recommended amount of aerobic and strengthening exercise.[36]

Yet it doesn't take much to meet these physical-activity guidelines for adults sixty-five and older:

- Get at least 150 minutes a week (30 minutes, five days a week) of moderate-intensity activity, such as brisk walking, *or* 75 minutes a week (25 minutes, three days a week) of vigorous-intensity activity (such as jogging or running); *and*

- Do muscle-strengthening activities two or more days a week for all major muscle groups (legs, hips, back, abdomen, chest, shoulders, and arms); *and*

- Do exercises that maintain or improve balance, if you are at risk for falling.[37]

> A common reaction to many of life's changes—including getting older—is to stop moving. Yet one of the best ways to maintain vitality and slow down age-related decline is to keep moving.

Yoga practice clearly meets many of these guidelines. The government's Centers for Disease Control and Prevention classifies yoga as a moderate-intensity activity[38] and recommends the practice as a way to strengthen muscles and boost balance.[39]

Safely practiced, yoga can help combat the relentless pull of gravity on muscles and bones, and the wear and tear caused by decades of use. "Age and gravity are the tartar of our skeletal system, [and] yoga is like postural dental floss," says Matthew J. Taylor, a physical therapist in Scottsdale, Arizona, and a past president of the International Association of Yoga Therapists.[40] Just as we brush our teeth daily, he recommends doing two 5-minute yoga practices a day. Even a brief, daily practice can help older adults learn—and be able to maintain—good posture, he says, which can enhance comfort, balance, respiratory function, and mood.

While yoga meets—or exceeds—the public health mandate for regular movement, the practice offers much more than physical exercise. In addition to the well-recognized posture practice, yoga's toolbox also includes breathing and meditation practices, which can influence emotional states, as well as guiding principles designed to counter toxic emotions such as anger and hostility. When practiced with one or more other people, yoga may also help relieve loneliness and isolation, which can be detrimental to health. The noncompetitive, supportive, welcoming nature of the practice makes yoga an ideal vehicle for physical, mental, and spiritual health benefits.

Partnering with Your Health Care Provider

For most people, it's much riskier to be sedentary than to exercise—as long as the activity is appropriate for you. So if you're in good health, you may not need to consult your doctor about starting the Relax into Yoga program. But if you have any health issues and/or questions, it's wise to talk with your physician and/or physical therapist to make sure the practice is safe and appropriate for you.

To enhance your safety, we encourage you to answer these questions:

Have you ever been told that you have heart disease or high blood pressure, or that you've had a stroke?

Have you had any major surgeries?

Are you taking any prescription medications?

Are you currently under a doctor's care for a medical condition?

Have you had any serious illnesses or injuries?

If you answered yes to any of these questions, it is advisable to tell your doctor that you are planning to start a yoga practice consisting of gentle movements and breathing practices designed to enhance relaxation, boost strength and balance, and improve flexibility and function. Since some physicians don't know much about yoga (and may think it involves standing on your head) you might even show him or her this book and ask if there are specific movements or practices that you should modify or avoid.

CHAPTER 2

Yoga for the Perfectly Imperfect Body

A side effect of the numerous medical advances made in recent decades is the dramatic rise in the number of people living with chronic illness. Approximately 80 percent of older adults have at least one chronic health condition, and 50 percent have at least two.[41] And in addition to diagnosed disorders, a significant proportion may have a "silent" disease, such as heart disease or osteoporosis, that has no obvious symptoms. In fact, an estimated 35 percent of postmenopausal white women have osteoporosis but may not be aware that they have this bone-weakening disorder and are at increased risk of fracture[42] (see "Osteoporosis," page 29).

Yoga practice can—and should—be adapted to address any health challenges that may arise. Sometimes these adaptations may be temporary. For example, someone with a broken arm may need to eliminate postures that place weight on the arm; modify those in which the arm is extended or elevated; and switch to more lying-down postures, breathing, and meditation. This may be necessary just until the arm is healed, after which it may be possible to resume the original practice.

However, with some health challenges, including many of those related to aging—such as the onset of arthritis, osteoporosis, or hypertension—more lasting adaptations may be advisable. For example, someone with glaucoma may need to stop practicing handstands, and someone with osteoporosis may switch from doing forward bends with a round back and straight legs to doing them with a straight back (neutral spine) and bent knees (see "Healthy Body Mechanics," page 52). We have partnered with medical experts to get their recommendations about potentially risky movements. Their wisdom is integrated into our Relax into Yoga postures. Below are specific recommendations for the most common health conditions.

Heart and Circulatory Problems

Age is one of the most significant risk factors for all cardiovascular ailments. This includes coronary artery disease, which is the most common type of heart disease and the leading cause of death for both men and women in the United States, as well as numerous other cardiovascular conditions such as hypertension, congestive heart failure, arrhythmias, valvular disorders, and stroke. With advancing age, the elastic elements of the blood vessels are progressively replaced by more leathery, fibrous tissue.

In addition, progressive deposition of cholesterol plaque in the inner walls of the arteries—known as atherosclerosis, or hardening of the arteries—can also compromise blood flow to vital organs such as the brain, kidneys, and the heart itself. Loss of elasticity in the heart muscle can lead to symptoms of heart failure. Wear and tear on the blood vessels over time can lead to aneurysms and clots, while wear and tear on the heart valves can lead to narrowing and leaking.

Practicing Yoga if You Have Heart or Circulatory Problems

For the reasons mentioned above, we recommend that people with cardiovascular disorders communicate their interest in practicing yoga with their physician (see "Partnering with Your Health Care Provider," page 24).

In addition, here are some cautions:

- **Avoid holding your breath.** This can affect your blood pressure. In particular, avoid holding your breath while straining—a practice known as the Valsalva maneuver. This habit is common among weightlifters and can also occur in daily activities, such as lifting something heavy or straining while going to the bathroom.

- **Avoid any kind of forceful breathing.** Also avoid practices in which you feel that you are struggling for breath. Keep your breath flowing comfortably throughout your practice. Breathing practices that encourage a gentle suspension of the breath at the end of the inhalation and at the end of the exhalation may be fine, but check with your physician if you have any questions.

- **Avoid extremes.** This includes extreme movements, extreme exertion, extreme breathing practices, and extreme temperatures. All of these can strain the cardiovascular system.

- **Avoid dropping your head back.** Extreme cervical extension (bending your neck way back) may cause pain or dizziness—or in extreme cases a stroke. In back-bending postures lift your chest and your gaze, but be sure to maintain the natural curve in the back of your neck.

We offer these recommendations as ways to enhance for your practice:

- **Be sure to keep your breath flowing easily and comfortably.** Maintain an awareness of your breath. Recognize that your breathing can be a reflection of what's going on in your body and mind.

- **Build your stamina in a slow and steady fashion.** Strength, endurance, and flexibility can be cultivated progressively over time without overtaxing your system.

- **Be mindful of gravity's effect on the cardiovascular system.** This can include:

- *Feeling dizzy or light-headed* when you move quickly to standing from sitting or lying down. This is called *orthostatic* (or "postural") *hypotension* and is a form of low blood pressure that may last from a few seconds to a few minutes. Be sure to move slowly and carefully when getting up from lying down or sitting, and have a chair or something else to lean on if necessary.

- *Shortness of breath when lying supine* (flat on the back) for some people with cardiorespiratory issues. Elevating the upper body with a wedge or pillows may be useful.

- *Headache, breathlessness, or possibly a stroke* from an inverted position where the head is below the heart. Avoid head-down positions.

- *Overloading a compromised heart* with an excess of fluid from an inverted position in which the legs are elevated on a wall while the torso rests on the ground. For someone with congestive heart failure that results in a pooling of fluid in the ankles and feet, this popular Legs Up the Wall pose may flood a struggling cardiovascular system. Elevating the legs to a lower, less-extreme angle may be fine, such as placing your legs on a bolster or a chair. Consult your physician if you have questions.

- **Recognize side effects of medications.** Your yoga practice may be affected by medications you are taking if they produce side effects such as dizziness, altered exercise response, lowered resting heart rate, and muscle aches.

- **Maintain proper hydration.** Drink some water before your practice, as dehydration may result in fatigue, dizziness, and/or fainting.

- **Remember that relaxation is very important for cardiovascular health.** Don't underestimate the benefits of practicing being still and quieting your body and mind.

- **Be aware of the symptoms of a heart attack.** These can include chest discomfort, shortness of breath, nausea and vomiting, breaking out in a cold sweat, and unusual tiredness and/or pain in the back, shoulders, and jaw. Not everyone has the sudden, crushing chest pain often shown on TV, and older, female, or diabetic people having heart attacks may have no chest pain at all.[43] If you think you, or someone near you, might be having a heart attack, call 911. Acting fast can save your life, and every second counts.

Osteoporosis

The word "osteoporosis" means "porous bones" and is a disorder of impaired bone strength that results in skeletal fragility and increased fracture risk. Caused by an imbalance between the natural process of bone breakdown and bone formation, this bone loss generally occurs in women after menopause and in both men and women with aging. The longer you live, the greater your likelihood of developing osteoporosis—with the disorder affecting about 15 percent of women in their fifties and about half of all women in their eighties.[44] You are at greater risk for osteoporosis if you:

- *Are female*—women after menopause are three times more likely to develop the condition than men.[45] But osteoporosis does affect men, too, with men over fifty more likely to break a bone from osteoporosis than to get prostate cancer.[46]

- *Have a small, thin body frame*—particularly if you weigh less than 127 pounds or have a body mass index less than 21.[47]

- *Are taking certain medications*—including long-term use of steroids (such as cortisone and prednisone), SSRIs (such as Zoloft, Lexapro, and Prozac), and some cancer chemotherapeutic drugs.[48]

With the aging of the population, the prevalence of osteoporosis is expected to increase so that by 2020 one in two Americans over age fifty is expected to have or be at risk of developing osteoporosis of the hip; even more will be at risk of developing osteoporosis at any site in the skeleton.[49] Four out of every ten white women age fifty or older in the United States will experience a hip, spine, or wrist fracture sometime during the remainder of their lives.[50] And these fractures can have devastating consequences. For example, people who break a hip have a higher risk of dying during the first three months after the fracture than individuals of similar age who do not break a bone.[51]

> By 2020, one in two Americans over age fifty is expected to have or be at risk of developing osteoporosis of the hip; even more will be at risk of developing osteoporosis at any site in the skeleton.

Since osteoporosis has no obvious symptoms, it's possible to have compromised bones and not know it. In fact, many people learn that they have osteoporosis only after they break a bone. *Osteopenia* is the name sometimes given to low bone density that is not low enough to be called osteoporosis. People with low bone density are at higher risk for osteoporosis and are more likely to break a bone compared to people with normal bone density.[52] These conditions are diagnosed by a test called a DEXA scan that measures bone mineral density at the hip and spine. The U.S. Preventive Services Task Force recommends this testing for women ages sixty-five and older as well as younger women at increased fracture risk.[53] But not everyone who is eligible gets this test. And, surprisingly, two-thirds of vertebral fractures do not come to clinical attention.[54] This means it's common for people to suffer this kind of fracture either without pain or with pain that is misidentified—as a pulled muscle, for example—and not recognized as originating from a vertebral fracture.

Practicing Yoga if You Have Osteoporosis

Physical activity can enhance bone health, particularly weight-bearing exercise such as walking, and muscle-strengthening movement such as weight training.[55] Many yoga postures and practices can be extremely beneficial in maintaining or improving strength and balance as well as restoring function and relieving pain for people with compromised bone. Weight-bearing postures such as Chair pose and Plank pose may help strengthen bones, as can poses that move the body against resistance, such as a Yoga Push-Up. However, some common yoga poses should be appropriately modified because they have potential for significant harm. In particular, forward bending (spinal flexion) and twisting (rotation) can place large and compromising loads on the front of vertebral bodies[56] and are often implicated in vertebral fracture.[57]

Movements to Avoid

If you have osteoporosis, the National Osteoporosis Foundation advises *against* the following movements:

- Bending forward from the waist

- Twisting or bending the torso (trunk) to an extreme

- Twisting the torso (trunk) and bending forward when doing activities such as coughing, sneezing, vacuuming, or lifting

- Toe-touches, abdominal crunches, and sit-ups.[58]

Keeping your spine in proper alignment—with good posture and healthy body mechanics—puts less stress on the spine and is particularly important if you are at risk of fracture (see "Healthy Body Mechanics," page 52). Be aware, too, that sitting puts more strain on your spine than does standing or lying down. For this reason, you won't find seated forward bends, seated deep twists, or any floor-sitting poses in our Relax into Yoga postures. We have substituted safer variations that help build and maintain spinal strength and flexibility with reduced risk.

Here are our additional recommendations for safe alignment during your yoga practice:

- **Avoid rounding your spine in sitting or standing.** We do not present any such postures in Relax into Yoga. But if you are an experienced practitioner and want to adapt potentially risky poses to meet these guidelines, doing so would require changes such as *not* pressing your hands into the ground to strongly arch your back in Cat pose and *not* doing Downward-Facing Dog pose with a rounded low back.

- **Avoid twisting your spine forcefully and/or to the end of its range of rotation.** Again, we do no present these movements. However it's not uncommon for some yoga poses to twist your spine as far as it will go, *then* invite you to press your hands or arms against something to push your twist a little further. We advise against this "end-range rotation" and suggest keeping twists in midrange using a smooth quality of motion.

- **Avoid placing your body weight on your neck and/or shoulders.** This includes avoiding poses such as Headstand, Shoulder Stand, and Plow.

Movements to Invite into Your Practice

Be sure to follow these movement tips for a safer practice:

- **Keep your spine long.** This is especially important when doing twists. Extend up from the top of your head and keep your rotation in a moderate range, such as how you might turn to look over your shoulder when driving.

- **Keep your head on the ground when lying on your back.** Lifting the head up when doing supine postures creates the forward-flexing "abdominal crunch" action that is contraindicated. When you are ready to get up from lying down, be sure to roll over onto your side, then use the strength of your hands and arms to push away from the ground (see "Healthy Body Mechanics," page 52).

- **Hinge from your hips (not your waist).** Do this with any standing or seated postures that involve bending forward. Remember to tilt your pelvis forward and keep your spine long. Avoid rounding your back. In standing movements that bend your body forward, hinging from your hips and bending your knees can help you maintain proper spinal alignment.

- **Use a support.** Practice balance poses near a support, such as the wall or the back of a chair, if you feel unsteady.

- **Move with a smooth, relaxed quality of motion.** Avoid jerky or ballistic movement.

- **Consider lying down or standing rather than sitting to "take a load off" your spine.** Recognize that lying down places the least stress on the spine and may be the safest way to practice many poses if you have very compromised bone. (If you can't get down onto the floor, it's fine to do lying-down poses on your bed.) Standing with good posture is the next safest way to practice poses. Sitting places the most stress on the spine, so be particularly mindful of the recommendations above when doing seated poses.

Joint Problems and Arthritis

If any or all of your joints are achy or painful, chances are you have arthritis. In fact, the word "arthritis" means "joint inflammation" and refers to more than one hundred different diseases that affect the joints and tissues around the joints. The onset of symptoms can be gradual or sudden and typically involves pain and stiffness around one or more joints. Symptoms may come and go but generally persist over time. While arthritis can affect people of any age, including babies, the prevalence increases as people get older. Nearly half of people sixty-five and older report doctor-diagnosed arthritis.[59] A major cause of disability in America, arthritis frequently limits people's ability to perform everyday activities such as dressing, climbing stairs, and walking.

A generation ago, people with arthritis were told to rest and "save their joints." Unfortunately, that practice did more harm than good since, as we now know, inactivity causes joints to stiffen and unused muscles to atrophy. In recent decades, study after study has confirmed the benefits of physical activity for people with arthritis, and it's now clear that appropriate exercise can greatly improve the quality of life for people with arthritis—relieving pain and stiffness, improving function, and boosting mood.[60] It can also help manage other chronic conditions, such as obesity, that may affect arthritis and its symptoms.

Three of the most prevalent types of arthritis are osteoarthritis, rheumatoid arthritis, and fibromyalgia.

Osteoarthritis

Typically when people say they have arthritis they mean osteoarthritis, which is the most common form of arthritis and is generally related to aging, injury to a joint, and/or being overweight.[61] Sometimes called "wear and tear" arthritis, or OA, osteoarthritis is characterized by breakdown of the cartilage that covers the ends of bones in a joint. As the cartilage wears away, bones rub together, which can permanently damage the joint. It's possible to have osteoarthritis in just one joint—for example a knee that was injured playing football. It most commonly affects the larger joints of the body—the hips, knees, spine, and shoulders—on one or both sides.

Rheumatoid Arthritis

Sometimes called RA, rheumatoid arthritis is a systemic inflammatory disease that affects multiple joints on both sides of the body. While the cause is unknown, RA is an autoimmune disorder, which means the body's immune system attacks its own tissues.[62] It commonly affects the smaller joints—such as the fingers, wrists, feet, and neck—on both sides of the body. RA can begin at any age, although it often starts in middle age and is most common in older people.[63] Two to three times more common in women than in men, RA is associated with fatigue, prolonged stiffness, and joint deformity.[64] While there is no cure, medications may help slow disease progression, and appropriate physical activity may help decrease pain and reduce the risk of joint deformity.

Fibromyalgia

Sometimes considered an arthritis-related condition, fibromyalgia is not actually a form of arthritis because it does not cause inflammation or damage to the joints.[65] But like arthritis, fibromyalgia can cause pain and fatigue, and it can affect the ability to perform daily activities. Other common symptoms include sleep disturbance, headaches, irritable bowel syndrome, cognitive problems with thinking and memory (sometimes called "fibro fog"), and numbness or tingling of the hands and feet.[66] Most people with fibromyalgia are women diagnosed during middle age, however men and children can also be affected.[67] While the cause is unknown, disease onset may be associated with a stressful or traumatic event, repetitive injuries, or illness and may be related to problems with how the central nervous system processes pain.[68]

Physical activity—including muscle strengthening and aerobic exercise—has been shown to be beneficial for people with fibromyalgia, as has cognitive behavioral therapy and relaxation. In fact, people with fibromyalgia who participated in the Yoga of Awareness program developed by Kimberly and her husband, Dr. Jim Carson, experienced reductions in pain levels that were greater than the reductions typically seen with medications.[68]

Practicing Yoga if You Have Joint Problems or Arthritis

The American College of Rheumatology states that exercise should be an essential part of treatment for arthritis, noting that "people with arthritis who exercise regularly have less pain, more energy, improved sleep, and better day-to-day function."[70] Yoga offers similar benefits to a Western exercise program—including enhancing balance, boosting endurance, and strengthening and stretching muscles surrounding the joints, all of which can decrease pressure on the joints and relieve pain. In addition, yoga teaches many physical, mental, and emotional skills that can be profoundly helpful for people with arthritis, including relaxation breathing, mindfulness, learning to move with compassion, recognizing and changing harmful habits (such as breath holding and jaw clenching), and pacing activity with rest.

> **The practice of mindfulness meditation can be an important tool for self-care, since it can improve depression, fatigue, stress, pain, attention regulation, emotion regulation, memory, and more.**

If you have arthritis, it's helpful to work with a physical therapist who can design an individualized exercise program that takes into account the kind of arthritis, the affected joints, and your overall conditioning. Your physical therapist can be a helpful partner in answering any questions you have about starting or continuing a yoga practice.

We offer these cautions for modifying your yoga practice:

- **Recognize that sharp, immediate sensations may be possible warning signs.** If you experience sharp pain during and/or immediately following activity, it is likely a sign that something is not right, and you need to modify what you are doing. Also, if you experience pain in a joint, back off and modify your activity.

- **Learn to distinguish between sharp pain and dull pain or muscle soreness.** Recognize that, if you've been sedentary, you may feel some muscle soreness or dull pain the morning after doing a new activity. This is called "delayed onset muscle soreness" and comes from using your muscles in unaccustomed ways. It is generally a sign of strengthening that is an expected part of getting stronger and typically goes away within a few days.

- **Avoid adding excessive pressure to affected joints.** For example, if you have osteoarthritis in your knee, you may not want to put all your weight on that leg in a balance pose. Instead, you might keep the toes of the opposite foot on the ground or lightly touch a countertop with your hand. If you have RA in your hands, you may want to modify a posture that places your body weight on the hands (such as Spinal Balance pose) by using a prop that takes the weight off your hands or by bringing your forearms to the ground rather than your palms.

- **Do not bend affected knees too deeply.** In standing poses with one or two bent knees, such as Warrior 2, be sure that when you look down over your bent knee you can still see your toes. If you can't, you are likely putting too much extra pressure on the knee.

- **Be mindful of overstretching with RA.** The disease can cause joints to become loose and unstable, so stretching beyond what feels comfortable can cause problems. In particular, avoid flexing your neck forward with added weight (such as using clasped hands behind your head to pull your chin toward your chest), which can put damaging pressure on vulnerable joints in the cervical spine.

- **Recognize red flags: joints that are red, hot, and/or swollen.** These are signs of active inflammation, which means exercising that joint could lead to further damage. Rest is generally advised during arthritis flares; however, gentle range-of-motion exercise may be helpful. Talk to your health care provider about appropriate treatment, which may include medication, ice or heat, and supportive devices.

Here are some strategies to enhance your practice:

- **Ease into any activity.** Start slowly and progress gradually.

- **Remember to warm up your joints.** Move all the body's joints through their comfortable range of motion every day. This can be particularly important in preparing for weight-bearing postures, as it helps to lubricate the joints.

- **Let gravity work for—not against—you.** If a posture places pressure on an affected joint, consider turning the pose upside down or sideways, so the body is in a different relationship to gravity, taking weight off the joint. For example, do Child's pose or Pigeon pose lying on your back to take body weight off your knees and ankles, or do Downward-Facing Dog with your hands on the wall to take body weight off your shoulders, arms, and hands.

- **Focus on strengthening the muscles that support your affected joints.** Muscles serve as shock absorbers, so strengthening the muscles can help alleviate pressure in irritated joints.

- **Use props (such as blankets and chairs) to help "take a load off" your joints.** For example, lightly touching a wall or chair can help relieve pressure on an arthritic knee or hip.

- **Remember that relaxation cultivates ease.** Practicing relaxation can relieve muscle tension and decrease the pain response.

Joint Replacement

Certain joints that have been damaged by arthritis or other causes may be surgically removed and replaced with an artificial joint. This often occurs when the pain becomes so severe that it interferes with the ability to function. The surgery is performed most often on hips and knees but also can be done with shoulders, fingers, ankles, and elbows.[71] The modern hip replacement was pioneered in the 1960s and is now, along with knee replacement, among the most commonly performed operations in the United States.[72] An estimated 4.7 million Americans have undergone total knee replacement, and 2.5 million have had a total hip replacement.[73] The prevalence of these surgeries is higher in women than in men and increases with age.

Typically, people with joint replacements are given specific movement precautions by their surgeon and work with a physical therapist to regain full mobility of the new prosthetic joint during the postoperative period and recovery process. Specific precautions are related to the particular surgical approach—that is, whether the surgeon approached the joint from the front of the body or the back of the body. For example, people who have a hip replaced with an anterior approach are told to avoid hip extension, which means not extending the affected leg behind you or stepping backward with the affected leg. People who have had a hip replaced with a posterior approach are told not to bend their hip past 90 degrees, which is why patients are given a raised toilet seat to use during the recovery period. For both hip replacement approaches, people are advised not to cross their legs or ankles.[74] In general, these precautions are followed for about six months, but in some cases they may be in effect for longer.

People who have knee replacements are generally encouraged to walk as soon as possible, often using a support—such as a cane, crutches, or a walker—during the first few weeks after surgery. Gradual resumption of daily life activities is typically recommended. In time, many people with knee replacement are able to kneel—for activities like gardening as well as to do kneeling postures in yoga—although it can be helpful to kneel on a cushion or folded blanket for comfort.

Practicing Yoga if You Have Had Joint Replacement

If you have had a joint replacement, it is essential that you get clearance from your surgeon, along with any special instructions, before beginning or resuming a yoga practice. In most cases, postsurgery precautions will be lifted in time, and you will likely be able to do all—or most—of the Relax into Yoga postures.

Lung Disease

Chronic obstructive pulmonary disease (COPD) is an umbrella term for a group of progressive lung diseases that causes blockage to airflow and makes it difficult to breathe. The two main types are emphysema and chronic bronchitis, and some experts also include certain forms of asthma.[75] The main cause of COPD is long-term exposure to substances that irritate the lungs, which—in the United States—is typically cigarette smoke. Outdoor and indoor air pollution, occupational dusts and chemicals, and respiratory infections can also play a role. In 2011, COPD was the third-leading cause of death in the United States[76] and is most common among people over age sixty-five.[77]

More than half of adults with impaired lung function are unaware that they have a problem, since—at first—symptoms may be nonexistent or mild.[78] Often people mistake early warning signs, such as breathlessness and coughing, with normal aging. For this reason, lung disease is often not diagnosed until the condition is very advanced.[79] While there is no cure for COPD, early detection can allow intervention before major loss of lung function occurs. Treatments include medications, supplemental oxygen, and—in severe cases—lung transplantation. Removing exposure to the source of irritation—for example quitting smoking—is essential.

In people with COPD, the airways become swollen and narrowed, losing their elasticity and making it hard to get air out. This "trapped air" leaves less room for new, fresh air and can create a sense of physical and emotional struggle as breathing becomes more and more difficult. Feeling breathless can lead to anxiety, which can exacerbate breathlessness and sometimes lead to panic. Pulmonary rehabilitation can be a powerful way to help people with lung disease become stronger and better able to function by teaching proper breathing mechanics, exercises, and other strategies to help improve quality of life. These classes are often affiliated with a hospital or clinic and are generally led by a pulmonary rehab team that may include doctors, nurses, physical therapists, respiratory specialists, exercise physiologists, and dieticians who can create a program that meets your specific needs.

Diaphragmatic Breathing

Teaching healthy breathing mechanics is an essential part of pulmonary rehabilitation and is also a central aspect of yoga practice. Learning diaphragmatic breathing—sometimes called "abdominal breathing" or yoga "belly breathing"—can be a powerful way to help people with lung disease strengthen and learn to properly use the diaphragm, which is the main muscle of breathing. When people have COPD, it is difficult for them to breathe, so they often compensate by using muscles in the neck, shoulders, and back (sometimes called "accessory muscles of breathing") to try and move air in and out. Over time, practicing diaphragmatic can make breathing more efficient and less effortful.

While yoga breathing generally advises breathing in and out through the nose, breathing out through pursed lips can be extremely helpful for people with COPD, since this technique slows the breathing, improves the exchange of oxygen and carbon dioxide, and keeps the airways open longer to release more trapped, used air.[80]

A useful way to remember this approach is with the phrase *Smell the roses, blow out the candles.* Follow these steps to practice pursed-lips breathing:

1. **Breathe in comfortably through your nose.** Inhaling through the nose is important because the nostrils have tiny hairs that warm, moisten, and filter the air.

2. **Pucker your lips in an "O" shape and breathe out slowly through your lips.** Imagine you are blowing out a long row of candles on a birthday cake.

3. **Repeat.** Inhale through your nose, then exhale slowly through pursed lips. Keep practicing and, over time, see if you can make your out-breath two times longer than your in-breath. So if you inhale to the count of three, you'd exhale to the count of six.

Practicing Yoga if You Have Lung Disease

Since many people with lung disease take medications that may weaken their bones, it may be helpful to practice the guidelines for osteoporosis (see "Osteoporosis," page 29). In addition:

- **Avoid slouching.** Sitting and/or standing slumped forward can compromise your breathing.

- **Don't forget the importance of your exhalation.** Rather than striving to "take a deep breath," instead focus on enhancing your exhalation by using pursed-lips breathing to help your body release trapped air.

Be sure to:

- **Include plenty of time for restorative poses and relaxation postures.** Having a regular relaxation practice can be extremely useful, since the struggle to breathe can create physical, emotional, and mental tension and fatigue.

- **Practice the Three-Part Breath pattern.** See page 72. This exercise will enhance your breathing efficiency. Be aware of using your diaphragm to power your breathing. Notice if you allow your back and ribcage to expand as you inhale and to relax as you exhale. Try to keep your neck and shoulders relaxed as you do this.

- **Stretch out your neck, shoulders, and upper back.** These areas typically carry excess tension (see "Neck Release," page 74).

- **Try Professorial pose any time you feel anxious and short of breath.** To do this, stand with your arms supported by a high countertop or table—like a professor leaning on podium. This can help keep your posture erect and your ribcage lifted to support efficient breathing.

Chronic Pain

Unlike acute pain, which is a normal sensation that alerts you to possible injury and goes away when the underlying cause has been treated or has healed, chronic pain persists; it's often defined as daily pain for at least three months.[81] Older adults are at particular risk for chronic pain because many of the medical conditions common to aging—such as arthritis, cancer, osteoporotic fractures, and diabetic neuropathy—often involve persistent pain. In addition, injuries or accidents from earlier in life can continue to cause pain throughout the life span. In fact, chronic pain is considered a "meta-condition," which means persistent pain is a common symptom in many different types of illness; it is rapidly becoming a major public health concern. In 2011, the Institute of Medicine's special report, *Relieving Pain in America*, noted that chronic pain affects about 100 million American adults, more than the total affected by heart disease, diabetes, and cancer combined.[82]

Chronic pain involves a complex series of processes in the brain and central nervous system, and physicians often have a difficult time offering ways to fully manage pain. Medications, such as opioids, may help chronic pain but are habit-forming with potentially serious side effects—such as drowsiness and impaired judgment, constipation, nausea, and itching. Opioids also require increased doses over time to maintain their effects, which can lead to accidental overdose deaths.[83] Surgical procedures are not always effective and sometimes can make things worse.

Recent neuroscientific research offers insight into why traditional pain treatments like drugs and procedures often have limited success. Despite the outdated belief that pain experienced is directly proportional to the injury suffered, new studies show that pain is strongly influenced by a broad array of other dimensions of experience, including thoughts, emotions, and movement patterns.[84] For example, emerging evidence indicates that negative emotions such as anger and fear can increase the experience of painful sensations and that positive emotions can dampen the pain signals in the central nervous system.[85] This is why programs that aim to change behaviors, thoughts, and feelings—and increase coping strategies—seem to hold the most promise for managing chronic pain. Yoga and meditation are examples of such programs.

> It is important to move your body to break the vicious cycle of inactivity that occurs with persistent pain.

Practicing Yoga if You Have Chronic Pain

The yoga practice's focus on moving mindfully and with compassion can be a helpful way to break the vicious cycle of inactivity that is common to people with chronic pain. Reintroducing gentle and appropriate movement back into your daily routine is an important step in changing this cycle. Using postures that improve strength and range of motion can help enhance vitality and boost your ability to function.

Yoga's focus on the breath is also an important tool for people living with persistent pain, and learning to use the breath skillfully can be a powerful tool in finding relief. It is common to discover that you hold your breath when you are under stress. Breath holding is a typical stress reaction that interferes with your body's ability to quiet itself and relax. The yoga practice develops an awareness of the breath and encourages fluid patterns of breathing. Learning breath patterns, such as the three-part diaphragmatic breath, also cultivates deeper states of relaxation, which can help dampen pain signals. Breathing in rhythm with the yoga movements can help settle your nervous system. Setting the intention to invite your breath to soothe a painful area can also have healing effects. Although clearly lung tissue only exists within the rib cage, studies demonstrate that the simple act of bringing attention to different parts of the body—for example, "breathing into your lower back"—increases blood flow to these areas.[86]

Another therapeutic aspect of the yoga practice that is important for living with persistent pain involves generating a shift in your relationship to the pain sensation itself. For many people this is an unfamiliar practice. When the body is experiencing persistent pain, a typical response is to tense the muscles and to consciously or unconsciously consider this painful sensation the "enemy." As part of yoga's "self-study" principle, people with chronic pain may learn to reconceptualize the experience as "sensation" rather than "pain" and practice accepting rather than reacting to the painful sensation—recognizing that acceptance is not giving up but simply being willing to have the experience you are already having. Over time, practicing acceptance can help the body and mind learn to quiet the reactivity to the experience and begin to shift the neurological wiring that occurs with chronic pain.[87]

The meditative practices of yoga can also help to ease persistent pain. Bringing awareness to the inner dialogue and commentary that constantly go on in the thinking mind can reveal "habits of mind" that may be exacerbating the pain experience. *Catastrophizing*, or the tendency to anticipate the worst possible scenario, is one such "habit of mind." Catastrophizing is not uncommon in people with chronic pain and is known to worsen the pain experience.[88] For example, thoughts like *This pain is going to destroy all my plans for the future*, or *This cursed pain has ruined my life*, or *It is not worth the effort to try and get better, nothing ever changes* can all contribute to heightening the intensity of the sensation. Deepening our awareness of our inner experience through yoga practice can help develop a perspective that doesn't give so much credence to such habits of mind. A deep awareness can also assist with being able to choose inner dialogue that is more supportive of healing. Recognizing that no one can predict the future and that what is happening in this moment is simply what is happening in this moment has the real potential of reducing suffering.

Likewise, being able to recognize our present-moment emotional response to pain can be a powerful tool. Although anger, sorrow, frustration, and fear are normal responses to pain, if these become emotional habits they can increase the level of pain that we feel. Being aware of the coming and going of the emotions without getting stuck in one particular emotion is a skill that can be developed with yoga practice.

Before beginning a yoga practice, older adults with chronic pain may want to check with their physician or physical therapist to determine whether a particular movement is appropriate (see "Partnering with Your Health Care Provider," page 24). Remember that it is important to move your body to break the vicious cycle of inactivity that occurs with persistent pain. Also, *when areas of your body have been in persistent pain, it will be unlikely that you can avoid pain.* So the common yoga directive "If it hurts, don't do it" may not apply. Instead, be aware that if a posture increases your pain significantly during or immediately after the movement, you will need to modify or omit this posture.

If you have chronic pain, be sure to:

- **Practice smaller movements at first.** Slowly build up to the larger movements. For example, if lifting your arms all the way over your head feels like too much, try bringing your arms just to shoulder height at first. This way you can work toward the larger movement with patience and compassion.

- **Pace yourself.** Practice by doing a little, resting for a short while, and then doing a little more.

- **Become friends with your breath.** Recognize when you tend to hold your breath, and use the Three-Part Breath pattern (see page 72) to invite ease.

- **Set the intention of bringing breath into painful areas.** Then see what you notice.

- **Pay attention to your inner dialogue.** While you are practicing, notice the thoughts in your mind. Recognize that these are just thoughts and that they are not you.

- **Do your best to soften out of any negative or judgmental thoughts.** Try to avoid fueling the negative commentary.

- **Practice self-compassion and kindness.** Recognize that acceptance is not giving up—it's being willing to have the experience you are already having. Letting go of resistance can relieve suffering.

Cancer

Cancer is considered a disease of aging because the older we get, the greater our chances of developing cancer become. The incidence of cancer in people over sixty-five is ten times greater than in those younger than sixty-five, and the cancer death rate is sixteen times greater in patients over sixty-five compared to younger patients.[89] Treatments have also advanced to a degree that cancer survivorship is more and more common, with an anticipated 19 million cancer survivors in the United States by 2024.[90] Some survivors experience very little ongoing effects of treatment, while others may struggle with troublesome side effects—such as fatigue, neuropathy, and lymphedema—for many years.

Practicing Yoga if You Have Cancer

Fortunately, a yoga practice can be adapted to help people navigate any phase of the cancer journey, from diagnosis through treatment, survivorship, and/or progressive disease. Each phase of the cancer experience brings with it various struggles and dis-ease in the body. By learning the benefits of various yoga practices, yoga can be an ideal supportive-care choice.

The initial diagnosis can be overwhelming and frightening. Facing the unknown of the stage and aggressiveness of the disease, as well as the possible outcomes, can lead to high states of anxiety and many sleepless nights. Yoga's Three-Part Breath pattern (see page 72) can be helpful in settling the body when awaiting results of surgical reports and lab work. Likewise, the postures help the muscles release the tension that can build up during this difficult time.

Treatments for cancer—which include surgery, chemotherapy, and/or radiation—are often quite challenging for the body, mind, and emotional heart. Nausea, fatigue, pain, and weakness are common side effects that can be difficult to mitigate. Yoga provides simple ways to help the body through this rough patch. For example, studies have demonstrated that diaphragmatic breathing can provide pain-relieving effects[91, 92, 93, 94] and improve sleep disturbance and anxiety in cancer patients receiving chemo.[95] Yoga practices have also been shown to significantly reduce chemotherapy-induced nausea and vomiting[96] as well as treatment and/or disease-related pain.[97]

Further, even in the difficult context of undergoing cancer treatments, it remains important to continue moving the body. Movement helps maintain a basic degree of physical fitness, which can help offset the debilitating effects of deconditioning that occur when the body is sedentary for long periods of time. In addition, physical activity can invigorate the body as well as facilitate subsequent relaxation. The gentle, mindful movements of the yoga practice are well suited to introduce movement in this phase of the cancer experience.

Mindfulness meditation practices can also support healing for older adults dealing with cancer. Studies of cancer patients demonstrate that the practice of mindfulness can improve quality of life, anxiety, depression, fatigue, sleep disturbance, stress, pain, cancer-related sexual dysfunction, physiological arousal (for example, blood pressure), immune function (immune cell count, cytokine production), and cortisol levels.[98, 99] In addition, studies of changes in brain structure and function suggest that mindfulness meditation helps with attention regulation, emotion regulation (especially capacity to calm fear), body awareness, learning, cognition, memory, perspective taking, empathy, and compassion.[100, 101, 102, 103, 104] The practice of mindfulness meditation can be an important tool for self-care.

As with any serious medical condition, people with cancer are advised to seek advice from their health care provider to ensure that their yoga practice is appropriate. (See "Partnering with Your Health Care Provider," page 24.) It's also advisable to:

- **Keep encouraging all of your body's joints through their full range of motion.** Do this even if there is tightness from scarring. This is important to regain and maintain optimal physical function.

- **Honor your energy levels.** Do not exercise to exhaustion. Balance periods of movement with periods of rest.

- **Have a sturdy chair nearby for support.** Do this when exploring standing postures if your balance is challenged, for example by neuropathy in the feet, fatigue, or weakness.

- **Follow the guidelines presented for osteoporosis.** This is important if you have decreased bone mass from cancer treatment or have lesions in your spine. (See "Osteoporosis," page 29.)

- **Wear a compression sleeve.** Do this when practicing these postures if you have swelling from lymphedema.

- **Use your own mat or make sure mats are properly cleaned to reduce risk of infection.** This is particularly important if you join a community class and your immune function is weakened due to treatments.

CHAPTER 3

Yoga for the Functional Body

If you're like many people in our computerized, sedentary world, you spend many hours crunched forward over computers, smartphones, and tablets. Even if you're engaged in domestic activities, like cooking, knitting, or rocking a baby, or yard work, like digging or planting, your focus is generally forward and your body tends to round in response. The all-too-common result of spending so much time hunched over laptops, steering wheels, and desks is rounded posture, which frequently becomes even more stooped with age. This "crunched forward" posture can compress internal organs and is associated with a wide array of ailments, including back and neck pain, breathing and circulatory difficulties, headaches, joint pain, and digestive problems.

A yoga practice can relieve these issues by helping people bring their bodies back into healthy alignment. This often requires stretching tight muscles and strengthening weak ones, enhancing joint flexibility, and learning proper body mechanics—including how to stand, sit, move, and lie down in ways that support optimum health. Benefits are enhanced when you take these teachings off the mat and into your daily life—for example, being sure to sit and stand with good posture throughout your day.

Healthy Body Mechanics

Try these healthy body mechanics basics on and off the mat.

Getting Down and Up from the Floor

The ability to get down and up from the floor is a key life skill that unfortunately many older adults lose—often through lack of practice and getting out of shape. It's not uncommon for people in their seventies and eighties to come to our yoga classes and tell us that they can't do postures lying on the floor because they haven't been on the floor in years. Often they'll say, only half joking, "I can get *down* onto the floor, but I won't be able to get back *up*." We always invite these folks to do postures sitting in a chair, and in our classes it's common for some people do postures sitting in a chair while others do them lying on the ground. Over time, some of these people learn how to get down and up from the ground and find the experience empowering. Depending on your physical limitations, however, it may not be advisable to try to get down and up from the ground. This may be a topic to discuss with your health care provider, who might recommend working individually with a physical therapist.

For those who are interested and able, here are some guidelines to safely getting down and up from the ground:

- **Have a stable support nearby.** A chair, bed, or low table that you can lean on can help in making this transition. If you're using a chair or table, make sure it is either securely pressed against a wall or so heavy that it won't slide.

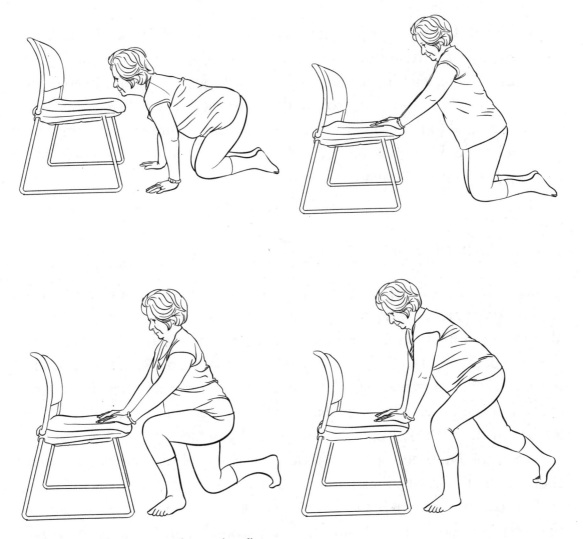

Figure 3.1 Getting up from the floor

- **To get up from down:** Lying on your back, bend one or both knees and roll onto your side. Use the strength of your hands and arms to roll over into an all-fours position. "Walk" on hands and knees to your chair, then place one hand and then the other onto the chair seat. Bring one knee forward, placing that foot on the ground. Use the strength of your legs—and the support of your core muscles and arms—to rise as you bring your back leg forward and come to standing (see figure 3.1). Be sure to take your time, since it's not uncommon to get dizzy when going from lying down to sitting or standing.

- **To get down from up:** Stand in front of the support, bend your knees, stick your bottom out, and place your hands securely on the support. Extend one leg back. Bring one knee to the ground, then the other (feel free to place something soft under your knees if you like). Then bring one hand to the ground, then the other, so you are on "all fours" (refer to figure 3.1, but in reverse order). From this all-fours position, lower yourself onto your mat.

Standing and Sitting

A popular yoga saying is "You are as young as your spine," and much of the yoga posture practice is devoted to cultivating strength, flexibility, and proper alignment of this structural and energetic core of our bodies. Extending from the back of the head to the pelvis, the spine consists of a column of cylindrical bones, known as vertebrae, which are stacked on top of each other like a string of pearls. Each vertebra has a solid part in front called the "vertebral body" and a space in the back that provides a protected passageway for the spinal cord. Together, the brain and spinal cord form the central nervous system, which coordinates the activity of all parts of the body.

In between each vertebra is a disc, a pad of cartilage with a jelly-like center that acts as a shock absorber and facilitates spinal movement. With age, the discs and vertebral bodies typically undergo degenerative changes that can contribute to stiffness and pain in the back and neck.[105, 106] Bone loss with age can also lead to vertebral fractures that result in a stooped posture, which can exacerbate pain and disability (see "Osteoporosis," page 29). For these reasons, keeping the spine in proper alignment—during yoga practice and in daily life—is essential to preventing and relieving pain and reducing the risk of vertebral fracture.

The spine is organized into four regions:

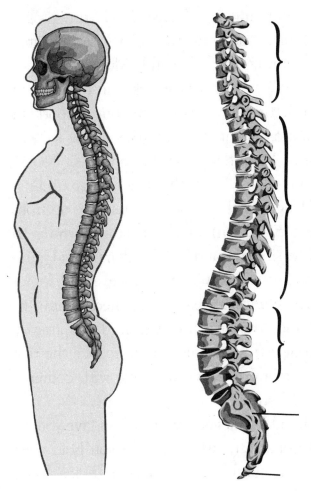

Cervical: Seven cervical vertebrae support the neck.

Thoracic: Twelve thoracic vertebrae connect to the ribs.

Lumbar: Five lumbar vertebrae support the lower back.

Sacral: The sacrum is a triangular bone at the base of the vertebral column consisting of five fused, modified vertebrae. At the bottom of the sacrum is the coccyx, which is sometimes called the "tailbone."

Figure 3.2 The spine

The common postural instruction to "stand up straight" is well-intentioned (since slumping is unhealthy) but inaccurate. A properly aligned spine is not actually straight but has four natural curves that give it strength and resilience, offering a springlike action that cushions the body from impact. From a side view, the cervical spine at the top and the lumbar spine at the bottom each curve toward the front of the body, while the thoracic spine and the sacral area each curve toward the back. From a side view, in a properly aligned spine, the ear is directly over the shoulder, and the shoulder is directly over the hip. This is a *neutral spine.*

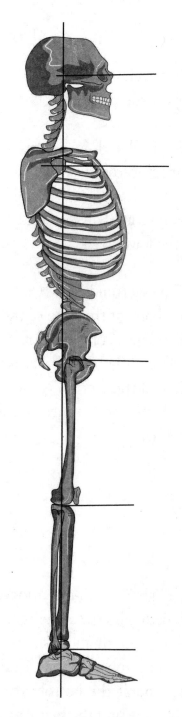

Figure 3.3 Neutral spine

Yoga's Mountain poses (both the seated and standing variations) teach the proper alignment of a neutral spine (see "Seated Mountain," page 106, and "Mountain Pose," page 90). In both postures, the focus is on first getting grounded from your support: in Standing Mountain pose this is the feet, in Seated Mountain pose this is the "sit bones" of the pelvis. From this place of grounding, we lengthen the spine by extending up from the top (crown) of the head. Learning to always sit and stand "tall" with a neutral spine is one of the best ways to relieve and sometimes eliminate back and neck pain, to enhance the health of the cardiorespiratory and digestive systems, and to reduce the risk of vertebral fracture in people with compromised bone.

In addition, good posture can give you an emotional lift, since the way you hold your body affects the way you feel, and vice versa. People who carry themselves with good alignment seem confident and graceful, while those whose posture reflects a physical slump often appear to be in a mental slump as well. Emerging research supports this notion, with one study showing that adopting an upright, seated posture in the face of stress can maintain self-esteem, reduce negative mood, and increase positive mood compared to a slumped posture.[107]

Bending, Lifting, and Carrying

A common movement often implicated in back injury and in vertebral fracture is bending forward from the waist with a rounded back. Adding weight to this movement—such as picking up a laundry basket or small child—puts even more load on the spine and increases the risk. That's why practicing good body mechanics—maintaining a neutral spine when bending forward, lifting, and carrying—is essential.

To do this, instead of rounding your back and bending forward at your waist, learn to keep your spine neutral, bend your knees, and hinge forward at your hips. An essential component of this action is identifying the "hip hinge," which is located at the crease where your thigh connects with your torso (trunk). Follow these steps to practice good forward-bending body mechanics:

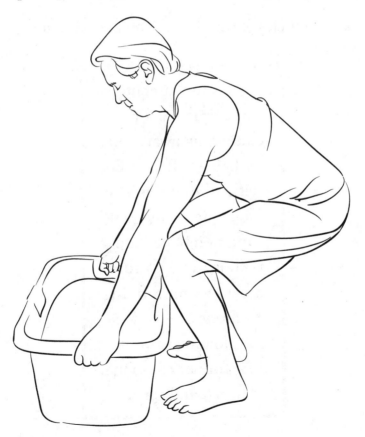

Figure 3.4 Lifting with good body mechanics

1. Place the pinkie-finger side of your hand in the crease where your leg meets your torso.

2. Keeping the natural curves in your spine, bend your knees and fold forward at your hips so that your body slightly squeezes your pinkie finger. (An excellent way to practice this motion and enhance the strength of your legs is by doing Chair pose; see page 94.)

If you are bending forward to pick something up, be sure to:

- Point your toes toward the object you will be lifting (to avoid twisting your spine with the added weight of whatever you're lifting). Then bend your knees and hinge forward at your hips with a neutral spine.

- Pick up the object and bring it in close to your body.

- Use the large muscles of your legs to come to standing.

> **Yoga is fundamentally a practice for cultivating awareness, for being fully present with all that arises in your life in an open and nonjudgmental fashion. The postures are a tool for refining awareness of what is unfolding in your body, mind, emotional heart, and spirit.**

Self-Study

Paying attention to your habitual patterns of movement and learning to replace risky motions with good body mechanics is an example of the yogic practice of *svadhyaya*, or "study." One of five self-disciplines outlined in the classic text *Yoga Sutras of Patanjali*, *svadhyaya* refers both to the study of sacred texts as well as to self-study. Rather than mindlessly moving through life, yoga asks us to be present, pay attention, notice that which is harmful (movements, attitudes, behaviors, and so forth) and instead choose that which is supportive. Self-study is central to self-understanding and, ultimately, to transformation.

If, like many people, you tend to live from the neck up, yoga practice can help take you out of your head and into your body, allowing you to identify any places of tension, tightness, or discomfort and—hopefully—learn to invite ease. Practicing the art of welcoming whatever arises, even if it's something difficult—such as a physical or emotional pain—can be essential to finding freedom from suffering. This is particularly important with the inevitable changes of age. Yoga breathing, postures, meditation, and principles can be essential tools to aging well—with vitality, grace, and joy.

PART 2

Relax into Yoga Practices

"We are all just walking each other home."

—Ram Dass

CHAPTER 4

Practice Guidelines and Essentials

The word "yoga" means "union," and the practice is designed to help us remember the connections among our mind, body, and spirit. It's also meant to bring us into union with our deepest, truest self. In contrast to the busy, outward focus of daily life, yoga practice invites us to slow down and turn our attention inward, to move mindfully and listen deeply to the quieter wisdom of our inner life.

Just as you would prepare for a reunion with friends and family, you will want to carefully attend to the details that will make your experience smooth and enjoyable. It's important to recognize that, unlike Western exercise, yoga is noncompetitive and does not involve strain. In fact, a central intention of yoga is to cultivate steadiness and ease. Here are some guidelines that can make your practice—this reunion with your self—steady and comfortable.

Prepare Your Space: Inspiration, Steadiness, and Comfort

You don't need fancy equipment, a large space, or expensive clothing to practice yoga. Any area in your home that is big enough for you to stretch out your arms and legs on the ground (or in bed) will do.

When we enjoy and feel comfortable doing something, we are much more likely to do it again. This is also true with yoga—so set up your space to best support an enjoyable practice. Pick a spot with a comfortable temperature. If the room is too hot or too cold, it will be less enjoyable, and your body will have to work harder to warm or cool itself. If there is a beautiful window you would like to practice in front of, time your practice so that the sun is not overheating the space.

Set up your practice space with an eye toward safety and comfort. For many older adults beginning a yoga practice, having a chair or a wall nearby can be useful for balance. We all have days when we feel steadier on our feet than others. The chair or the wall can provide great support on those wobblier days. If coming up and down from the ground isn't something that you have done in a while, a chair can be a particularly helpful tool for reclaiming this important life skill.

You might also want to have a few props nearby to make your practice more comfortable. Many people like to use a yoga "sticky" mat, especially if they will be practicing postures on the ground. A folded blanket or pillow can be helpful to cushion your head or knees if necessary. A strap can make some of the postures that stretch the legs more comfortable. But you don't need to buy a special strap; a bathrobe tie or a necktie can work quite well.

As your yoga practice will be a precious time for nourishing your body and steadying your mind, you might enjoy placing one or more special, inspiring objects in your practice space. For example, a photograph of a loved one or favorite pet, a treasure from a special trip, or even a fresh flower can reinforce for you why it is important to continue practicing. These reminders of afternoons with a grandchild, walks with a beloved pet, or time in your cherished garden may be a strong motivator for keeping your body and mind as healthy and functional as possible.

Prepare Your Body: Inside and Out

The yoga practice asks us to use our bodies and minds in new and sometimes unfamiliar ways. To prepare for these challenges, make sure you are well hydrated and nourished. However, it is not recommended that you practice directly after eating. Allow your body a couple of hours to digest a full meal, and thirty to sixty minutes to digest a small meal, prior to practicing the postures. Drink some water and, if you like, have a light snack—such as a piece of fruit or glass of milk—before practice. For people living with diabetes, monitor your blood sugar and eat a snack if necessary before beginning a yoga session.

As it doesn't feel great to practice with a very full belly, consider practicing first thing in the morning just after you wake up or before lunch or dinner. Some people enjoy a gentle practice in the evening before bed. If you choose this end-of-day rhythm, you might want to focus on relaxing, simpler poses, since some of the stronger postures can be quite invigorating and may make falling asleep more difficult.

Wear comfortable, nonrestrictive clothing. And to reduce the risk of falls—as well as to stretch and strengthen your feet—we recommend practicing barefoot. If you need the support of shoes as you are developing your practice, that is fine. However, it is not advisable to practice in your socks, as they are quick to slide, especially on tile, wood, or other smooth-surfaced flooring. If you have cold feet or prefer to wear socks for any other reason, invest in a pair of yoga socks, which have gripper dots on the bottom and separate each individual toe.

Always check in with how your body is feeling overall. If you feel stiff or sore, allow time for a slow warm-up before moving on to more challenging postures. If you are fatigued, try some gentle stretches and relaxation, and then see how you feel—you might be surprised at how invigorating a simple practice can be.

Prepare Your Mind: Intention, Awareness, and Connection

Just like you might set a resolution at the new year to take better care of yourself or be more available for your loved ones, you can set an intention for each practice session. In the yoga tradition, *sankalpa* is the term used to describe such resolutions or intentions. We suggest setting the intention to stay present—so that if you find your mind wandering off during your practice, you will do your best to bring your attention back to the present moment.

> Yoga is a practice of awareness designed to quiet your mind and help you connect with your innermost self.

Yoga, as it has been passed down through the ages, is fundamentally a practice for cultivating awareness, for being fully present with all that arises in your life in an open and nonjudgmental fashion. The postures are a tool for refining awareness of what is unfolding in your body, mind, emotional heart, and spirit. For example, deepening your relationship to the sensations in your body can be helpful in recognizing when patterns of tension or stress first arise. Or you may notice that certain emotional responses arise in reaction to a particular posture (that is, fear when feeling unsteady in a balance pose or frustration when encountering a physical limitation). As your practice deepens, you will become better and better at recognizing when the commentary in your mind is causing additional stress in your body and be able to make more skillful choices.

Many of us have habits of multitasking, reactivity, and distractibility. Yoga can shed light on these habits of heart and mind, so maintaining a steady and disciplined practice can help you learn healthier ways of being.

We recommend practicing the postures *at least* three times a week and the breathing practices daily. Even if you only have ten minutes to practice, it is better to do a little practice than no practice.

Please recognize that yoga is not just about training your body—you are also training your mind. So during your yoga practice, when you notice you are thinking about what you will have later for dinner or how a difficult conversation went earlier, simply notice the tendency of your mind to lose focus. Without judgment or frustration, redirect your attention to your breath and/or to the sensations of your movements. Likewise, if you experience a strong emotional current, see if you can stay steady by trying to simply *feel* the feeling without trying to explain it, force it to go away, or change it. Just feel how it feels in your body, then see what happens. Remember: steady and comfortable is the intention.

In addition to helping you stay present in the moment, focusing attention on your breath can also be a powerful tool for staying steady and comfortable by alerting you to times when you cross the line from challenge into strain. If you find yourself holding your breath as you practice a posture, or if your breath becomes ragged or shallow or compromised in any way, it may be a sign that you are doing too much and should back off the pose until you can breathe comfortably. Let your breath be your teacher, giving you insight into what is true for you in this moment.

Prepare Your Practice Rhythm: Steady and Comfortable Buildup

The Relax into Yoga program is designed to ease you into a regular yoga practice during the course of six weeks, and we recommend that you make a commitment to practice regularly so that you can enjoy the full benefits yoga can offer. During the first week, you will learn the foundational skills of the Three-Part Breath, the Range-of-Motion Sequence, and Relaxation pose—all of which are described in chapter 5 (week 1).

During each of the following weeks, please begin each practice session with the Three-Part Breath, then warm up with the Range-of-Motion Sequence. Next, you'll try a new sequence each week ("Standing Poses to Enhance Strength and Balance" in week 2, for example, and "Seated Poses to Improve Alignment, Flexibility, and Strength" in week 3). Be sure to finish each practice session with Relaxation pose. This approach will incorporate some practices that are familiar and some practices that are new each week. At the end of the six-week exploration, you will have experienced dozens of postures and have a good sense of how they work in your body, and the ways in which they support your daily activities.

As you build your practice, it is helpful to also begin incorporating brief mini-practices into your daily life. For example, try to:

- Bring your attention to your breath when you are waiting at a red light.

- Become aware of your posture when you are standing in the checkout line.

- Notice the commentary running in your mind before sleep and shift your attention to the sensations in your body instead. This can be particularly helpful if you are having difficulty sleeping.

> **Integrating yoga's teachings into your daily life encourages your practice to become even more vibrant and supportive.**

This approach to practice is sometimes referred to as "yoga off the mat." Integrating yoga's teachings into your daily life encourages your practice to become even more vibrant and supportive.

CHAPTER 5

Week 1: The Foundational Practice to Relieve Tension and Enhance Flexibility

All of the foundational practices described for week 1 can be done either lying down on the floor or in your bed. This sequence is a simple, gentle warm-up for your body and mind, and can be used as a stand-alone practice or as a limbering-up practice for sequences introduced in later weeks.

Learning how to let go and be still is as essential as learning how to move.

Functional Benefits of the Foundational Practice

Releases tension. The Three-Part Breath exercise (see page 72) helps deepen and expand the breath, which can release tension-holding patterns that interfere with a fluid breath and help soothe the system.

Reduces risk of injury. Taking time to warm up all the major joints and muscles before a longer practice tunes us in to how the body is doing and may reduce the risk of injury.

Enhances flexibility of the spine. Gentle neck and spine rotations support our ability to perform many activities of daily living, including driving—as healthy rotation is essential to being able to back up a car and/or change lanes.

Encourages joint mobility. Taking each of the body's major joints through a full range of motion can help enhance and maintain joint flexibility and function.

Induces relaxation. The ability to learn to "undo" tension in your body, mind, and emotional heart offers your entire being a welcome opportunity for deep rest.

The practices in this chapter and the ones that follow are available as downloadable audio at http://www.newharbinger.com/33643.

Three-Part Breath

This breath pattern is an invaluable tool for giving your body and mind a quick reset by intentionally guiding your belly, ribs, and chest to expand on the inhalation and fully relax on the exhalation. Sometimes called "diaphragmatic breathing," it is often used therapeutically to reduce pain, anxiety, and sleep disturbance. The Three-Part Breath practice can be done anywhere and anytime, multiple times a day or at night. While you can do this practice in any position—lying down, sitting, or standing—it's easiest to learn when you're lying down or sitting in a reclined position. Try this breath for a few moments (5 to 7 complete rounds) and then notice how you feel.

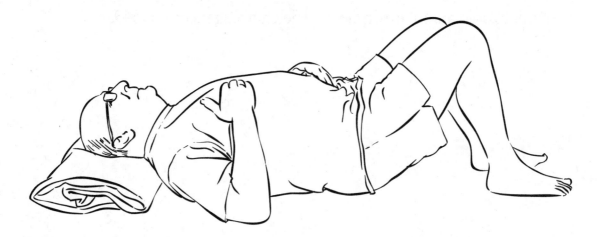

Figure 5.1 Three-Part Breath

Part 1: Rest your hands on your belly, just below the navel. As you take your next breath in, let your belly soften and expand like a balloon. As you breathe out, let your belly sink toward your spine. Repeat 3 times.

Part 2: Rest one hand on your ribs and one hand on your belly (see figure 5.1). With your next inhale, let your belly soften and feel your ribs expand to the left and to the right. As you exhale, let everything sink. Repeat 3 times.

Part 3: Rest the hand that was on your ribs on your upper chest, just below your collarbones. As you breathe in, allow your belly to soften, your ribs to expand, and your upper chest to broaden. As you exhale, let everything go. Repeat 3 times. Spend a few moments here, with one hand on the chest and the other on the belly, exploring this three-part rhythm. Allow this full, easy breath to open and nourish your body.

As you release the Three-Part Breath pattern, take a moment to notice how your body responded, how your emotional heart responded, and how your mind responded to this breathing practice.

Note: Three-Part Breath is *not* meant to be used all the time during your practice. It should be done as a periodic reset for your body and mind.

Range-of-Motion Sequence

Neck Release

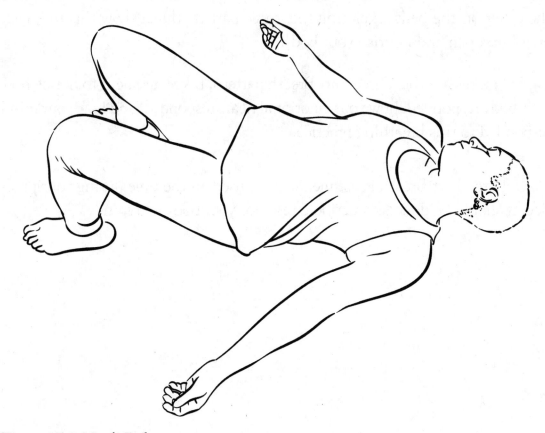

Figure 5.2 Neck Release

Setup

Lie on your back with your knees bent, soles of the feet flat on the ground, and arms at your sides. If your chin is higher than your forehead, place a folded blanket or towel behind your head so that your chin is at the same level—or slightly below—your forehead. Tune in to your breath.

Movement

Inhale in place.

Exhale and rotate your head to the right, looking over your right shoulder (see figure 5.2). Invite your left shoulder to be a little heavier.

Inhale back to center.

As you exhale, rotate your head to the left, looking over your left shoulder. Invite your right shoulder to be a little heavier.

Repeat this for a few cycles of breath.

Feel free to linger with your head rotated to the right and then left. Close your eyes, if you like, and feel into the sensations.

Remember

- Try not to force your head in one direction or the other.

- Be sure to keep the natural curve in the back of your neck. If you are elevating your head with a folded towel or blanket, make sure it's not so high that your neck flattens.

- Notice, without judgment, any differences between the movement to the right and to the left.

Arms Overhead

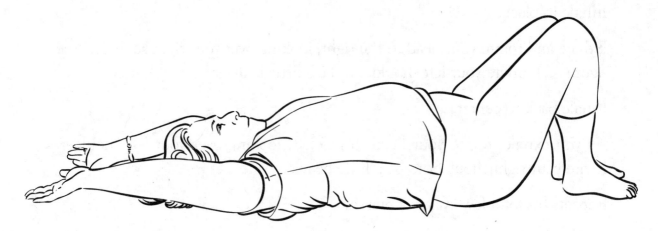

Figure 5.3 Arms Overhead

Setup

Lie on your back with your knees bent and the soles of your feet resting on the ground. Bring your arms alongside your body, palms facing down, and tune in to your breath.

Movement

As you inhale, extend your arms up and overhead so the backs of your hands move toward the ground behind you, or as close to the ground as they will comfortably go (see figure 5.3).

As you exhale, bring your arms back up and return them to the starting position, down along your sides.

Repeat for a few cycles of breath.

Remember

- Synchronize your movement with your breath so that your arms are moving toward your ears as you breathe in and toward your hips as you breathe out.

- Feel free to bend your elbows as much as you need to for comfort.

- Don't worry if the backs of your hands don't reach the ground. Just do the best you can without force or strain.

- Enjoy the feel of your breath.

- Take a moment to rest after you've finished, and try to notice any echoes of movement in your shoulders and arms.

Universal Legs

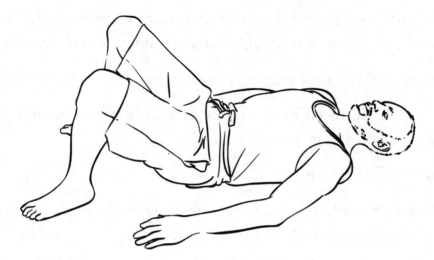

Figure 5.4

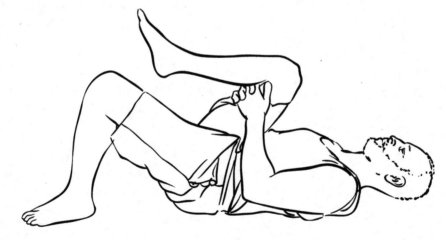

Figure 5.5

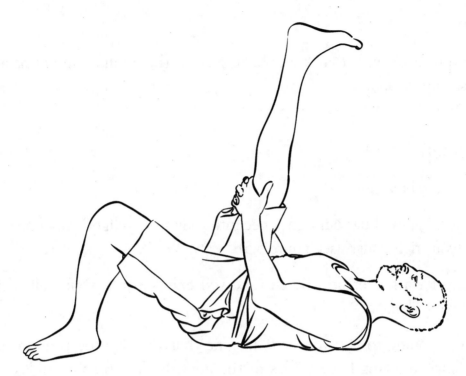

Figure 5.6

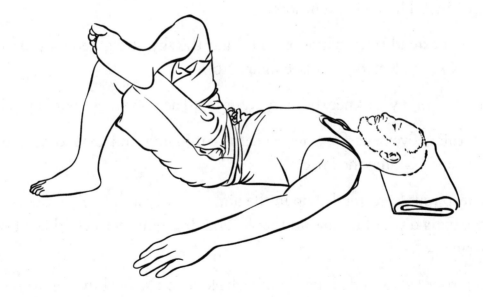

Figure 5.7

Setup

Lie on your back with your knees bent, feet on the ground, and arms at your sides (see figure 5.4).

Movement

Take an easy breath in.

On an exhalation, hug your right knee into your chest—lightly holding your leg behind your right thigh (see figure 5.5).

Stay here for a few breaths. Each time you exhale, draw your right thigh in toward your rib cage.

Next, continuing to hug your leg, imagine that your big toe is a crayon and begin slowly drawing large circles in the air to wake up your ankles. When you're ready, reverse the direction and draw a few more slow, easy circles going the other way. Then relax your foot.

Inhale and extend your right foot up toward the sky, straightening your leg as much as you comfortably can (see figure 5.6).

Exhale and bend your knee, bringing your foot back down by your buttocks.

Repeat this movement for a few breaths—inhaling and extending the leg, exhaling and bending the knee.

Next, keep your leg extended up in the air, with your leg as straight as is comfortable. Extend your foot toward the sky and drop your buttocks down toward the ground.

Keeping your leg extended, flex your right foot so the heel lifts up to the sky and the toes reach toward your nose. Then point your right foot, so your toes reach up to the sky.

Repeat this flexing and pointing a few times.

Relax your foot and draw big circles in the air with your toes, taking your ankles through their full range of motion. Circle a few times in both directions.

Next, bend your right knee and bring your right ankle onto your left thigh (see figure 5.7). Flex your right ankle to maintain healthy alignment in your knee. Linger here, bringing your attention to any sensations that arise and inviting your breath to soften any places where you feel tension.

When you are done, bring your right foot back to the ground, and rest here for a moment, relaxing and releasing. Notice if you feel any difference between your right side that you've just challenged, and your left side, which hasn't had a turn yet.

Now repeat the sequence with the left leg.

When you are done, release both feet to the ground, knees bent, and relax for a few easy breaths.

Remember

- If holding your leg is a strain on your shoulders or arms, use a strap behind your thigh to catch your leg, or rest your arms on the ground as you move your leg through the sequence.

- As always, challenge yourself, but don't strain—just do the best you can.

- Synchronize your movements with your breath—inhale as you straighten your leg, exhale as you bend your knee.

- Avoid holding your breath. Keep it flowing comfortably.

- Notice where you feel the sensation of stretch and movement.

- Notice where you feel the sensation of relaxing and releasing.

Supine Twist

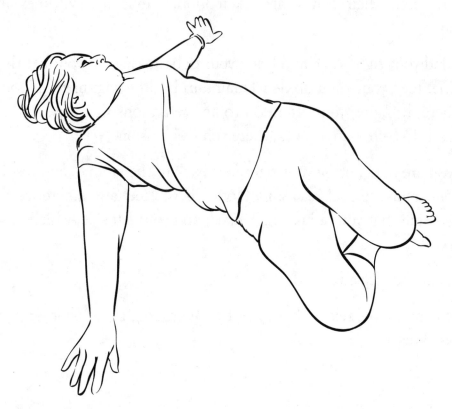

Figure 5.8 Supine Twist

Setup

Lie down with your knees bent and your feet about hip-width apart. Extend your arms out to the sides, palms up or down, whichever feels better.

Movement

Rock your knees from side to side, slowly and gently. Be sure to keep your feet on the ground.

Turn your head in the opposite direction of your knees, keeping your movement and your breath smooth and easy (see figure 5.8).

Repeat a few times.

Linger with your knees dropped to one side and your head rotated to the other. Rest here for a few breaths.

As you inhale, fill your body with breath. Inhale into your hips, waist, ribs, and armpits.

As you exhale, soften into the twist. Let each exhalation be an opportunity to release and let go.

When you are ready, inhale your legs back to center and square yourself off.

Then exhale and linger with your knees dropped to the other side. Rest here for a few breaths.

When you are done, come back to center with bent knees and both feet on the ground, and relax.

Remember

- When resting in the twist, feel free to place a rolled blanket or towel underneath your leg for support if your knee doesn't comfortably reach the ground.

- Do not force your leg to touch the ground.

- Release the weight of your arms and shoulders into the ground as you gently rotate your spine above and below this area.

Relaxation

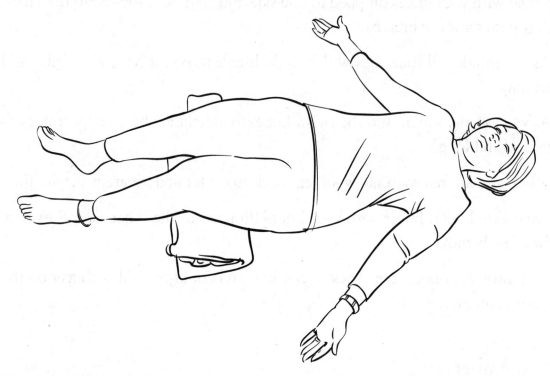

Figure 5.9 Relaxation pose

Setup

Rest with your legs straight or knees bent, whichever is most comfortable. Feel free to place a rolled blanket or towel under your knees. Let your hands relax by your sides, palms turned up or down, whichever position allows your shoulders to feel the most at ease (see figure 5.9). Close your eyes and give over the weight of your body to the ground.

Movement

Take a full breath in and let it go with a sigh.

Again, take a full breath in and release with a sigh.

One last time, take a full breath in and exhale with a sigh.

Become aware of the pool of sensation that is your body.

Feel the sensations of your feet, your legs, your pelvis, your torso, your hands, your arms, your shoulders, your neck, and your head.

Sense into your body as a whole, greet your body with kindness, and let it be.

Become aware of the waves of your emotional heart.

Sense the joy, the fear, the contentment, the anger, the sadness, the love.

Feel the currents of your heart all at once, greet your heart with kindness, and let it be.

Become aware of your thinking mind and the tendencies of your thinking mind.

Recognize the remembering, the forgetting, the liking, the disliking, the comparing, the evaluating, and the creativity.

Notice all of the tendencies of your thinking mind at once, greet your thinking mind with kindness, and let it be.

For now, the invitation is to simply *be*.

Remember

- The "undoing" is as important as the doing—learning how to let go and be still is as essential as learning how to move. Give yourself plenty of time for relaxation.

- Consider setting a timer for 5 or 10 minutes—or however long you want to practice Relaxation pose—so you can completely surrender to the experience.

CHAPTER 6

Week 2: Standing Poses to Enhance Strength and Balance

As you progress to week 2, hopefully the foundational practices from week 1 are feeling more familiar. Continue using the Range-of-Motion Sequence to prepare your body for the more-demanding strength and balance poses you will be learning this week. Your practice will follow this outline:

Begin with the Three-Part Breath exercise.

Warm up with the Range-of-Motion Sequence.

Explore the Standing poses in this sequence.

Finish with Relaxation pose.

Physically, standing poses help strengthen our legs, keep us grounded, and ease our ability to navigate a sometimes challenging environment. Metaphorically, these postures help build confidence, teaching us how to stand firmly on our own two feet.

> The standing poses give us practice in forming healthy habits on and off the mat, like hinging from our hips and bending our knees to keep length in our spine, rather than rounding our back forward.

Functional Benefits of the Standing Practice

Builds strength. Standing poses build dynamic strength, which can help maintain fitness for demanding activities, such as picking up your favorite toddler, walking your dog, and carrying grocery bags.

Establishes good body mechanics. The standing poses give us practice in developing healthy habits, like hinging from our hips and bending our knees to keep length in our spine rather than rounding our back forward. Also, learning to use the larger muscles of the thighs and buttocks to power our movements, rather than the smaller muscles of the back, is a "back-saving" technique that can be applied to various daily activities, from lifting a basket of laundry to getting in and out of a car.

Improves posture. Standing with good alignment offers stability, helps us radiate confidence, and enhances our ability to move through the world with ease.

As a reminder, you can download audio for week 2's practice at http://www.newharbinger.com/33643.

Mountain Pose

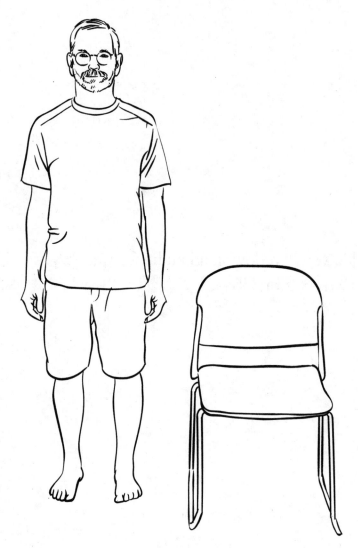

Figure 6.1 Mountain pose

Setup

Stand beside or behind your chair, close enough to lightly touch the back of the chair for support, if needed. Position your feet hip-width apart and snuggle the soles of your feet into the ground.

Movement

Energize your legs, as if you were drawing up energy from the ground.

Release your tailbone down toward the ground, lengthening your lower back.

Gently draw your lower belly in and up, and lift your rib cage up off of your pelvis.

Relax your shoulders down away from your ears, and allow your arms to rest by your sides.

Extend the top of your head up toward the sky, so that your spine elongates.

Let you chin be parallel to the ground, neither lifted nor tucked.

Gaze softly toward the horizon, with your shoulders, throat, and face relaxed (see figure 6.1).

Let the light of your heart shine forward.

Take several slow, easy breaths, filling and emptying your lungs completely.

Remember

- Feel yourself as strong and stable as a mountain.

- Sense the simultaneous downward and upward energies: rooting your legs and lifting your spine.

Salutation Arms

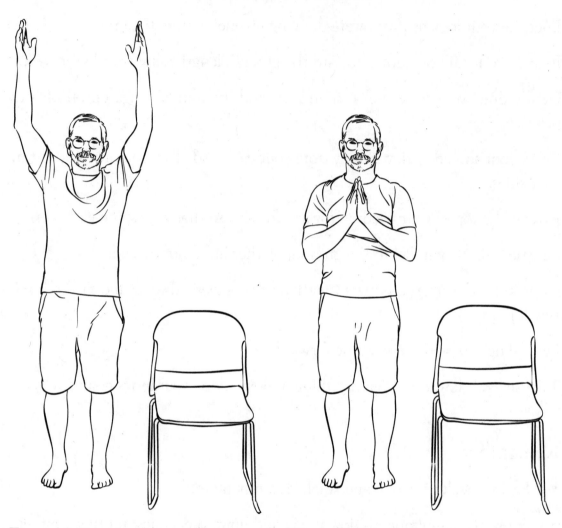

Figure 6.2   **Figure 6.3**

Setup

Stand beside or behind your chair in Mountain pose.

Movement

Inhale as you lift your chest, rotate your palms out, and extend your arms out to your sides. Lift your arms only as high as your ears.

Exhale and turn your palms down as you lower your arms, standing tall.

Repeat a few times.

Next, inhale your arms out to the sides and then up toward the sky as far as comfortably possible (see figure 6.2).

Exhale as you bring your palms together and lower them into a prayer-like position in front of your chest (see figure 6.3).

Repeat several times, moving with the breath. Imagine that you are gathering energy on your inhale and bringing the energy to your heart on your exhale.

When you are done, pause to take a few breaths with your palms touching and the base of the thumbs at your breastbone.

Remember

- Take this movement to a place that feels challenging but is not a strain.

- Synchronize your movements with your breath.

- Keep your shoulders as relaxed as possible throughout this practice. If you have restricted motion in your shoulders, feel free to lift your arms only slightly and/or modify the movement to suit your body.

- Notice the quality of sensations that are present.

- Notice the quality of emotions or thoughts that are arising. Try to simply let them be.

Caution

- If you need to hold on to the chair to feel stable, try lifting one arm at a time.

- You can also try this practice with your back against a wall for support.

Chair

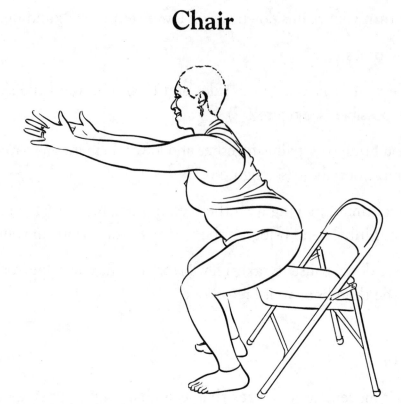

Figure 6.4 Chair pose

Setup

Make sure your chair is firmly grounded on a nonskid surface, preferably against a wall if it is a lightweight chair. Stand in front of your chair, so that the backs of your legs are an inch or two in front of the chair. Come into Mountain pose with your feet hip-width apart and parallel to each other.

Movement

Place the pinkie-finger side of your hands in your hip creases—the spots where your legs meet your torso.

Inhale and lengthen up through the top of your head.

Exhale as you bend your knees and hinge forward at your hips—keeping your spine long—while you extend your arms forward (see figure 6.4) and slowly lower yourself into the chair.

Inhale as you sit tall in your chair.

Exhale and root into the ground with your feet as you hinge forward at the hips and return to Mountain pose.

Repeat a few times. As your strength builds, try lingering with your bottom just above the chair seat—hovering in Chair pose without actually sitting down for several breaths—and then return to standing.

When you are done, return to Mountain pose.

Remember

- Be sure to draw your bottom back far enough so that you can see your toes when you hinge your hips and bend your knees. This helps to keep length in your spine as well as to keep pressure off your knees.

- The hip hinge is a very important anatomical landmark for learning how to lean forward without rounding your upper back, which is particularly significant for those with compromised bone.

- This practice is very strengthening for the quadriceps—the muscles in front of your thighs. They are called the "muscles of independence" because the ability to get up and down from a chair is a crucial skill for being able to live independently.

Caution

- This pose can feel rather demanding. Make sure you do not hold your breath.

- If your knees are tender or particularly painful, you may want to try the "as if" version of Chair pose (see page 118).

Warrior 2

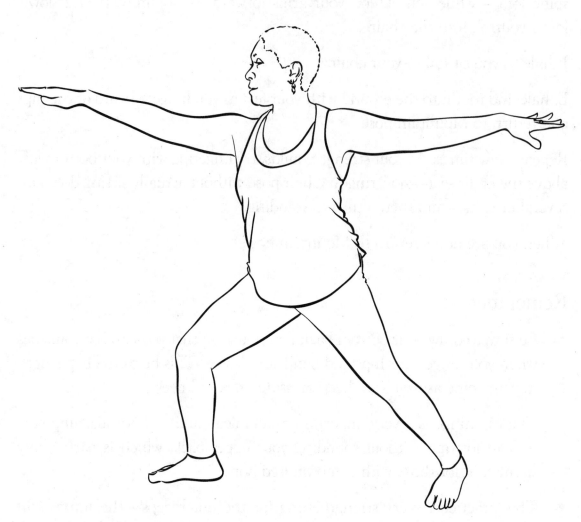

Figure 6.5 Warrior 2 pose

Setup

Stand behind your chair with your legs in a wide stance.

Movement

Rotate the toes of your right foot 90 degrees to the right.

Rotate the toes of your left foot about 15 degrees or so to the right. Gently root into your left heel.

Inhale and extend your arms out to your sides while lengthening your spine upward.

Exhale and bend your right knee until it is over your right heel and pointing in the same direction as the toes of your right foot.

Rotate your head to look out over the fingers of your right hand (see figure 6.5).

Inhale and straighten your right knee.

Exhale and bend your right knee.

Continue for a few breath cycles.

Linger in the bent-knee position for a few breaths if you like.

Repeat on the other side.

Remember

- Make sure you can see your toes when you bend your knee—avoid bending the knee so deeply that you can't see your toes.

- Keep your bent knee pointing in the same direction as the toes to avoid straining your inner or outer knee.

- Hold the chair lightly with one hand if you need support.

Caution

- This is a large-muscle activity and can be demanding. Please keep your breath flowing comfortably. Avoid holding your breath.

Side-Angle

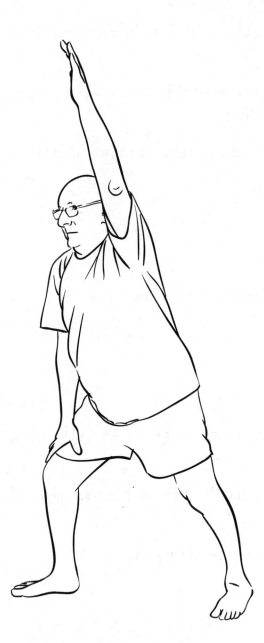

Setup

Stand behind your chair in a wide stance, as with Warrior 2 pose.

Movement

Rotate the toes of your right foot 90 degrees to the right.

Rotate the toes of your left foot about 15 degrees to the right. Gently root into the left heel.

Inhale and extend your arms to the sides while lengthening your spine upward.

Exhale and bend your right knee until it is over your right heel and pointed in the same direction as the toes of your right foot.

Keep your breath flowing as you place your right hand on your right thigh.

Extend your left arm toward the sky as high as is comfortable (see figure 6.6).

Figure 6.6 Side-Angle pose

Linger here for a few breaths. On each inhalation, allow your breath to nourish the entire left side of your body. On each exhalation lengthen your left side body, pressing down through your left heel as your reach up with your left hand.

When you are ready to come out of the pose, straighten your right knee, lower your left arm, and bring your body back to center.

Repeat on the other side.

Remember

- Make sure you can see your toes when you bend your knee over your heel.

- Keep your bent knee in line with your toes to avoid strain on your inner or outer knee.

- If you have the range of motion and strength, try placing your forearm on your thigh to deepen the stretch.

Caution

- This is a large-muscle activity and can be demanding—so please keep your breath flowing.

Triangle

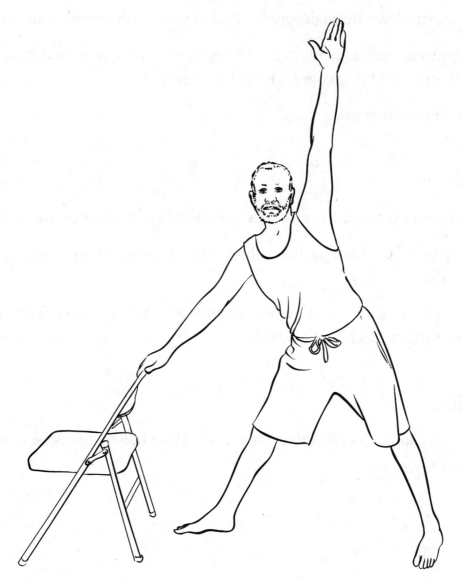

Figure 6.7 Triangle pose

Setup

Stand behind your chair in a wide stance, as with Warrior 2 and Side-Angle poses.

Movement

Rotate the toes of your right foot 90 degrees to the right.

Rotate the toes of your left foot about 15 degrees to the right. Gently root into your left heel. Keep your legs straight, but don't lock your knees.

Inhale and extend your arms to the sides while lengthening your spine upward.

Exhale and root into your feet as you tilt your torso to the right, keeping both sides of your torso long and your legs straight.

Lengthen your right arm toward your right leg. Let your right hand rest on the chair for support, if you like.

Extend your left arm either out to the left or up toward the sky (see figure 6.7). Keep your gaze forward, keeping the front and back of your neck long.

Linger here for several breaths, keeping your breathing steady and inviting any tense places to soften.

To come out of the pose, relax your arm down and bring your body back to center.

Repeat on the other side.

When you are done, come to Mountain pose and notice what arises.

Remember

- Keep both legs straight during this posture. It's fine to let your knees be soft and not locked.

- Be sure your top shoulder does not droop forward toward your chest. Feel broadness in your collarbones.

- If the shoulder of the lifted arm is tensing toward the neck, invite your shoulder blades to come together in the back of your body to bring softness and ease to the base of your neck.

CHAPTER 7

Week 3: Seated Poses to Improve Alignment, Range of Motion, and Strength

Most of us spend the vast majority of our days sitting down—often with poor posture. Slumped sitting can be a major contributor to back and neck pain and can also negatively impact breathing, circulation, digestion, and bone health. This chapter teaches healthy sitting alignment, which can help bring ease during your practice and throughout your day. The practices introduced here are also important tools for enhancing your ability to move your joints through a normal, pain-free range of motion, which can be a determining factor in your ability to live an independent, vital life.[108] Remember to start with the Three-Part Breath exercise, warm up with the Range-of-Motion Sequence, and finish with Relaxation pose.

> **Learning to always sit and stand "tall" with a neutral spine is one of the best ways to relieve and sometimes eliminate back and neck pain.**

Functional Benefits of the Seated Practice

Relieves back and neck pain. Sitting with a neutral spine can reduce pressure and pain in the back and neck.

Increases range of motion. Enhancing arm and shoulder mobility can increase our ability to reach things we want—whether it's an item on a higher shelf at home or in a store, or a tall loved one we'd like to hug.

Encourages fluid breathing. Articulation of the arms, shoulders, and spine can help improve breathing efficiency by reducing muscular holding patterns that interfere with a fluid breath.

Promotes independence. Strengthening the thighs is vital to being able to get up out of your chair, which is why the thighs are considered the muscles of independence.

Improves fine motor skills. Stretching and strengthening the hands and fingers can ease stiffness and increase suppleness, enhancing our ability to do activities that require fine motor skills, such as using a computer, cooking, and knitting.

Increases stability. Since our feet are our foundations for balance, stretching and strengthening the feet and toes enhances our stability, in addition to easing stiffness and decreasing foot pain.

As a reminder, you can download audio for week 3's practice at http://www.newharbinger.com/33643.

Seated Mountain

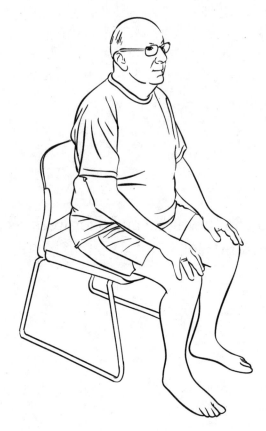

Figure 7.1 Seated Mountain pose

Setup

Sit slightly forward of the back of your chair, and place your feet on the ground, hip-width apart. If your feet don't reach the ground, use a folded blanket or towel to "raise" the ground to meet your feet.

Movement

Reach under your bottom to find your sit bones—those two hard "knobs" at the base of your pelvis.

Move the flesh away so that your sit bones can release down into the support of your chair.

Lift up from the top of your head, inviting your spine to lengthen up and your chest to lift a bit.

Relax your shoulders and your neck.

Keep your eyes forward with a soft gaze.

Rest your hands on your thighs or in your lap, wherever they are most comfortable (see figure 7.1).

Soften your face and release the hinge of your jaw, so your teeth gently part and your lips barely touch.

Soften the inside of your mouth.

Breathe into the stability of the Seated Mountain pose. Linger here for three to five easy breaths, feeling the dual action of your sit bones releasing down into the chair and the top of your head lifting up toward the sky.

Remember

- It can be surprisingly demanding to sit without the support of the back of your chair. If you begin to fatigue, feel free to scoot your hips back to rest your back against the chair.

- You may also put a rolled towel between your spine and the back of the chair for a nice gentle support as you build the strength to sit without support.

- When we get tired, we tend to round forward and collapse the chest. Try to keep the center of your chest gently lifted.

Caution

- Sitting with the spine slumped forward can put excess pressure on vertebral bodies, which may be problematic for people with back pain and/or low bone density. Do your best to sit with good posture.

Finger and Toe Flings and Curls

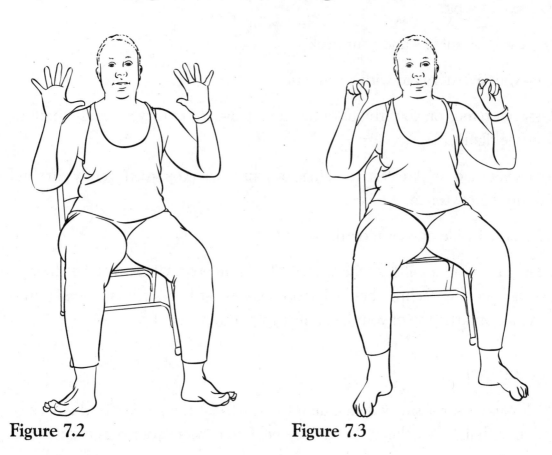

Figure 7.2　　　　　　　　**Figure 7.3**

Setup

Sit tall in Seated Mountain pose: sitting slightly forward of the back of your chair, feet hip-width apart on the ground (or a prop).

Movement

Bend your elbows and open your hands wide—palms facing forward.

Curl your fingers into a soft fist—make sure there is no tension in your hands, arms, or shoulders.

Inhale and fling your fingers open.

Exhale and make a soft fist.

Repeat several times.

Shake out your hands and rest them on your lap.

Keep your heels on the ground, but lift the tops of your feet up.

Fling out your toes, seeing if you can spread them wide so no toe touches another toe.

Fist your toes, curling them in.

Continue with this a few more times. Sit tall and keep your breath flowing.

Next, spread your toes and, with your heels still grounded, move your feet side to side, as if they were windshield wipers.

Next, move your feet out and in.

Relax your feet, sit tall, and notice echoes of the movement.

Next, as you sit tall and keep your breath flowing, fling out your fingers and toes (figure 7.2), then fist your fingers and toes (see figure 7.3). Do this several times.

Next, fling out your right hand and right foot. Then fling out your left hand and left foot.

Next, fist your right hand and left foot. Then fist your left hand and right foot.

Shake them out and relax.

Breathe into the stability of Seated Mountain pose. Notice any echoes of movement.

Remember

- Keep your breath flowing. Avoid holding your breath.

- Notice the sense of invigoration in the feet and hands.

- Notice any thoughts that arise. How did your heart and mind respond to this playful practice? Just notice.

Infinity Shoulders

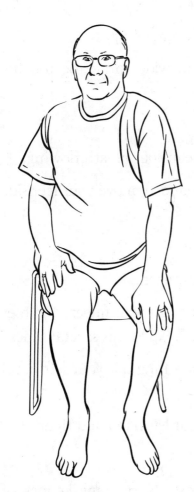

Figure 7.4

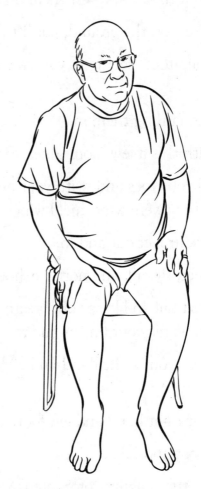

Figure 7.5

Setup

Sit tall in Seated Mountain pose: sitting slightly forward of the back of your chair, feet hip-width apart on the ground (or a prop).

Movement

Rest your hands in your lap.

Bring attention to the top of your right shoulder and lift it up toward your right ear as you drop your left shoulder down toward your hip.

Slide your right shoulder back as your move your left shoulder forward (see figure 7.4).

Drop your right shoulder down toward your hip as you lift your left shoulder toward your ear (see figure 7.5).

Bring your right shoulder forward as you slide your left shoulder back.

Explore making this figure eight, or infinity loop, through your shoulder girdle for several cycles, moving slowly and keeping your breath easy.

Next, change directions for a few cycles.

When you are done, pause and simply notice your experience here and now, sitting in stillness.

Remember

- Notice where the body feels tight and where it feels more fluid.

- Try pausing in a particularly tight or sticky place, and welcome breath into that area.

- Stay present as the subtler sensations fade and the body integrates the experience.

Universal Arms

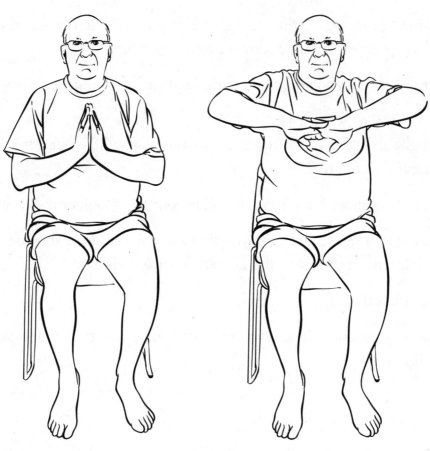

Figure 7.6   **Figure 7.7**

Setup

Sit tall in Seated Mountain pose: sitting slightly forward of the back of your chair, feet hip-width apart on the ground (or a prop).

Movement

Bring your palms together in front of your breastbone (see figure 7.6).

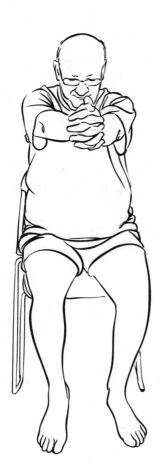

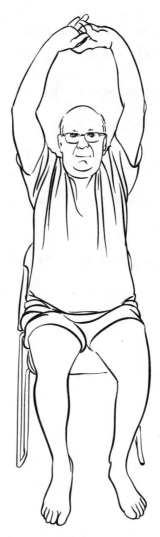

Figure 7.8

Figure 7.9

Pause and feel your breath.

Interlace your fingers.

Inhale and float your elbows up toward the sky (see figure 7.7).

Exhale and turn your knuckles forward as you extend your arms forward, dropping your head toward your heart (see figure 7.8). Be sure to keep your chest lifted—not collapsed—as you do this.

Inhale and turn your palms away from your chest, keeping your fingers interlaced, as you extend your arms up toward the sky (see figure 7.9).

Exhale and sweep your arms out to the sides.

Inhale as you bring your palms together in front of your breastbone.

Exhale as you interlace your fingers.

Repeat the sequence two or three more times, synchronizing your movement with your breath.

When you are done, pause in Seated Mountain pose and rest in the wave of the breath.

Remember

- Sit tall with a neutral spine and relaxed shoulders.

- Notice the response of your body.

- Notice the waves of sensation.

- Notice the currents in your heart.

- Notice any reflections in your mind.

Side Bending

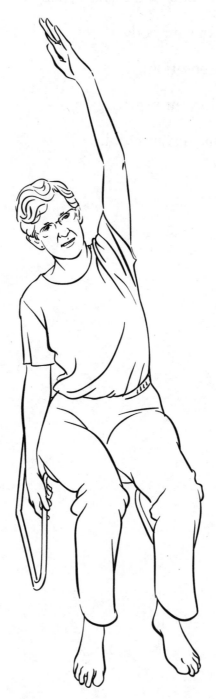

Figure 7.10 Side Bending pose

Setup

Sit tall in Seated Mountain pose: sitting slightly forward of the back of your chair, feet hip-width apart on the ground (or a prop).

Movement

Sit tall and tune in to your breath.

Let your right arm hang by your right side.

Inhale your left arm out to the side and up toward your ear, rotating your arm so your palm faces in.

Exhale and tilt your torso to the right (see figure 7.10).

Balance the weight evenly in the left and right buttocks.

Breathe into the left side of your body.

Inhale the left arm back toward the sky as you bring your torso back to center.

Exhale and sweep the left arm down to rest in your lap.

Repeat on the other side.

When you are done, come back to Seated Mountain pose and rest here for a few breaths.

Remember

- Avoid letting the raised arm collapse forward toward the chest.

- The lifted arm can extend out to the side if that is more comfortable for the shoulder.

"As If" Chair

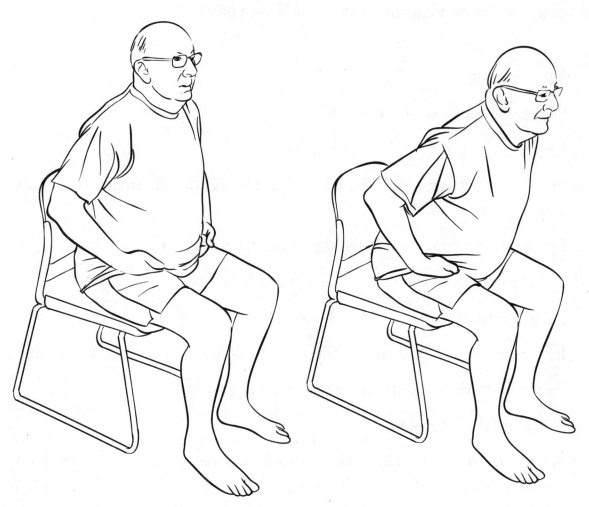

Figure 7.11   Figure 7.12

Setup

Sit tall in Seated Mountain pose: sitting slightly forward of the back of your chair, feet hip-width apart on the ground (or a prop).

Movement

Sit tall and tune in to your breath.

Bring your hands to your hip hinges, the place where your legs meet your torso (see figure 7.11).

Inhale and lengthen your spine.

Exhale and root firmly into your feet as you hinge slightly forward at your hips (see figure 7.12). Be sure to keep your spine long and your chest lifted.

Activate your body as if you were going to come to standing.

Inhale as you return your spine back to an upright position and relax your legs.

Explore taking your body through this movement "as if" you were going to stand. Repeat several times.

Remember

- Feel your thighs, lower legs, and buttocks enliven then relax.

- This practice builds thigh strength, which can be very important in maintaining function and independence.

- If you choose to come to a standing position, root your feet into the ground and use the strength of your legs to come up and out of the chair. Keep your chest lifted and avoid rounding your back. It is best to work toward being able to stand up from a chair using the strength of your legs rather than needing to use your arms.

Hugging Arms

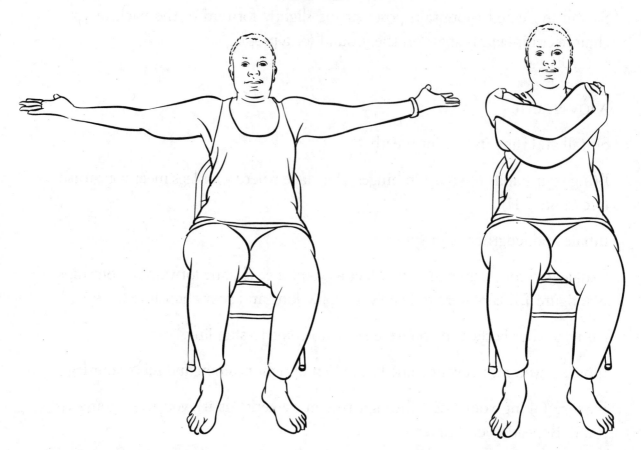

Figure 7.13   **Figure 7.14**

Setup

Sit tall in Seated Mountain pose: sitting slightly forward of the back of your chair, feet hip-width apart on the ground (or a prop).

Movement

Sit tall and tune in to your breath.

Inhale your arms out to your sides at shoulder height.

Exhale and relax your shoulders, keeping your arms extended and parallel with the ground.

Inhale as you rotate your palms up and "spread your wings," extending your arms farther out to the sides (see figure 7.13).

Exhale and cross your left arm over your right as close to your chest as is comfortable.

Keep your breath flowing as you wrap your hands around your upper body and give yourself a hug (see figure 7.14).

Soften your shoulders and gently twist your upper body by rotating slightly to the right and left.

Return to center.

Explore lifting your elbows up off your chest and then releasing the elbows down.

Return to center.

Keeping your chest lifted, let your head relax down toward your heart.

Breathe into the back of your neck, upper back, and shoulders.

Return your head to the starting position.

Inhale and uncross your arms, reaching them out to the left and right.

Exhale your arms down to rest in your lap. Linger here for a few breaths and notice how this feels.

Repeat this entire sequence, this time crossing your right arm over your left.

Remember

- Keep the twists gentle. Do not force your body into its maximum rotation.

Seated Backbend

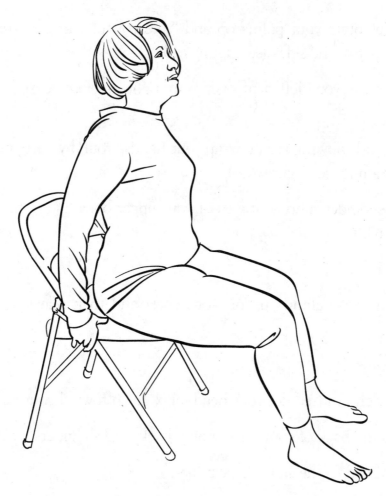

Figure 7.15 Seated Backbend

Setup

Sit tall in Seated Mountain pose: sitting slightly forward of the back of your chair, feet hip-width apart on the ground (or a prop).

Movement

Sit tall with your hands holding the seat of the chair behind your hips.

Lengthen your spine from your tailbone all the way up to the crown of your head.

Shrug both shoulders back and down.

Inhale and lift your breastbone toward the sky.

Exhale and slide your shoulder blades toward each other as you continue to lift your chest.

Let your gaze extend up, but be sure to keep both the front and back of your neck long (see figure 7.15).

Take a couple of easy breaths in this seated backbend position, then release back to sitting tall.

Explore this practice several times, then sit quietly and observe the effects.

Remember

- Notice how your body responds after the backbend.
- Notice how your emotional heart responds.
- Notice how your mind responds.

Caution

- Do not drop your head back. Keep the length in the back of your neck.

CHAPTER 8

Week 4: Balance Poses to Boost Strength and Reduce Fall Risk

Continuing to challenge and build our ability to balance is important across the life span, especially as many older adults find that balance worsens with time. Metaphorically, staying balanced in the midst of life's various challenges requires many frequent, small adjustments. The qualities necessary to balance in yoga postures—getting grounded, finding your center, staying focused, and steadying your mind—can also help you stay balanced in life.

Maintaining the ability to balance can decrease your risk for falls, which are the number-one cause of fractures, hospital admissions for trauma, loss of independence, and injury deaths in older adults.[109] The practices introduced in this chapter are designed to help build your strength and enhance your balance.

> **The qualities necessary to balance in yoga postures— getting grounded, finding your center, staying focused, and steadying your mind— can also help you stay balanced in life.**

Functional Benefits of the Balance Practice

Cultivates muscle memory. Intentionally introducing unsteady situations in which the body has to find its balance helps train the musculature that keeps the body upright.

Boosts spatial awareness. Balance postures can also refine our proprioception by strengthening the neurological pathways that tell us where our body is in space, boosting our ability to safely maneuver through our environment.

Enhances confidence. Seeing positive effects over time in your ability to balance can decrease both fear of falling and unnecessary activity restriction.

As a reminder, you can download audio for this week's practice at http://www.newharbinger.com/33643.

Tree

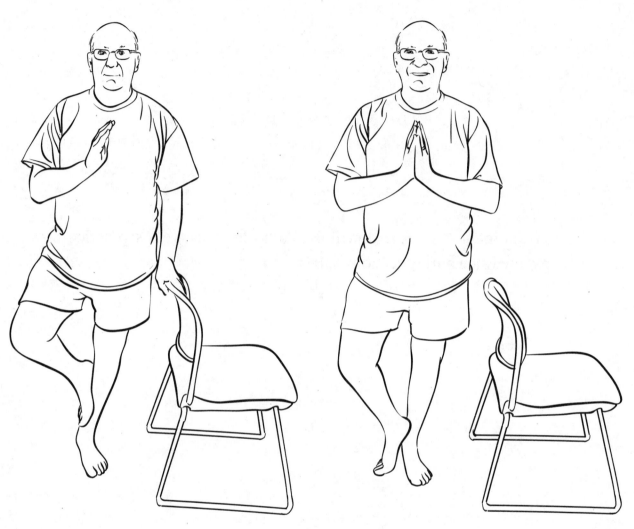

Figure 8.1   **Figure 8.2**

Setup

Stand beside your chair close enough to lightly touch the back of the chair for support. Position your feet hip-width apart, and snuggle your soles into the ground.

Movement

Stand tall in Mountain pose with your weight evenly distributed between both legs.

Send "roots" down through your right leg.

Lift your left heel, keeping the ball of your left foot on the ground.

Turn your left knee out slightly to the left as you slide the sole of your left foot against your right ankle.

Steady your gaze at the horizon and breathe easily.

For more challenge, pick your left foot up off the ground and place the sole anywhere along the inside of the right leg, except on the knee. Feel free to lightly hold the chair for support if you like (see figure 8.1).

Explore bringing your palms together in front of your chest. Feel free to touch your left foot back on the ground if necessary (see figure 8.2).

For even more challenge, extend your arms up overhead with your shoulders relaxed.

Play with balancing here for several breaths, then return to Mountain pose.

Repeat on the other side.

When you are done, stand in Mountain pose for several breaths and notice any thoughts, feelings, and physical sensations that arise.

Remember

- Breathe comfortably and observe the small adjustments required to maintain balance.

- Try to visualize yourself as a tree—are you a sturdy oak? A supple willow? A stately palm?

- Allow your breath to help your pose blossom from the inside out.

- Notice if you feel any difference between your ability to balance on each side.

Caution

- Avoid pressing your foot directly against the knee of your standing leg.

- Avoid locking or hyperextending the standing knee. Keep it "soft" by maintaining a slight bend.

- If the knee or hip of your standing leg is painful, practice keeping the toes of the bent leg on the ground to reduce the pressure on your standing leg.

Palm Tree

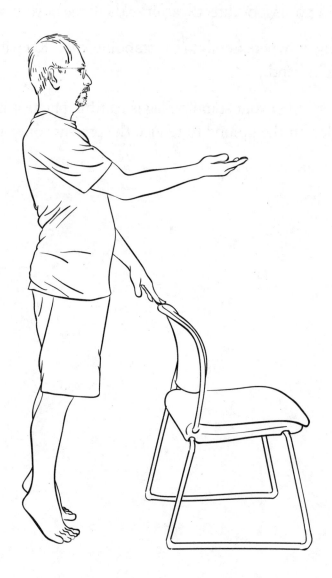

Figure 8.3 Palm Tree pose

Setup

Stand behind your chair close enough to lightly touch the back of the chair for support. Position your feet hip-width apart, and feel the ground beneath your feet.

Movement

Rest your fingers lightly on the chair.

Stand tall in Mountain pose with your weight evenly distributed between your legs.

Inhale and lift your heels up as high as comfortable, continuing to stand tall.

Exhale and lower your heels back down.

Repeat several times, synchronizing your movement with your breath.

For extra challenge, stay in the "up" position for a few breaths.

Explore moving one or both hands away from the support so that you're balanced on the balls of your feet (see figure 8.3).

To further challenge your balance, try extending your arms overhead.

After a few breaths, bring your heels back to the earth.

Remember

- Notice how your body responds to the balance challenge.

- Notice how your emotional heart responds to feeling unbalanced.

- Notice any comments in the thinking mind.

Caution

- If you are tall and have to stoop over to rest your fingers on a chair, practice with a wall as your support.

Warrior 3

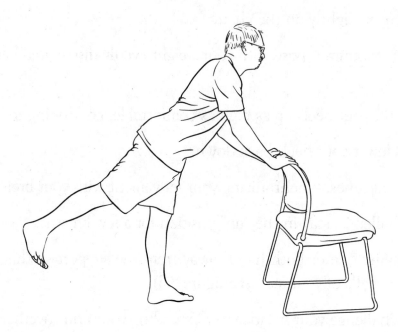

Figure 8.4

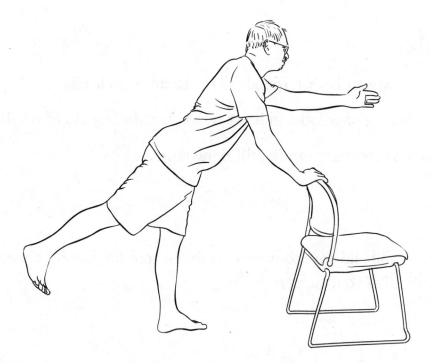

Figure 8.5

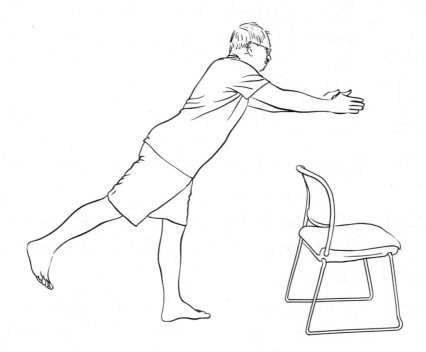

Figure 8.6

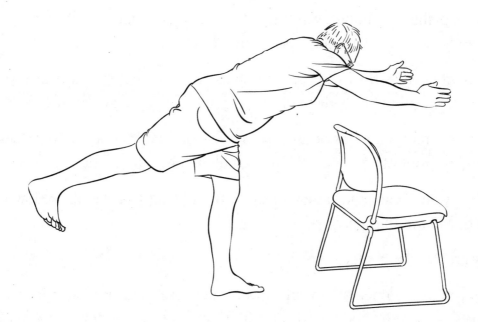

Figure 8.7

Setup

Stand behind your chair close enough to lightly hold on to the back of the chair for support. Position your feet hip-width apart, and feel the ground beneath your feet.

Movement

Rest your fingers lightly on the back of the chair and stand tall in Mountain pose.

Inhale as you lengthen up from the top of your head, then exhale as you hinge forward at your hips and slide your right leg back, keeping the toes and ball of the right foot on the ground.

Breathe comfortably in this position and, when you feel steady, float your back foot up away from the ground, keeping the back leg as straight as possible with the foot flexed (see figure 8.4). Keep the standing leg straight also, but don't lock your knee.

Explore moving one hand away from the chair (see figure 8.5). Try moving both hands away from the chair (see figure 8.6).

For more challenge, float the back leg up as you bow the torso forward so that your back leg and upper body are in a long line like a seesaw (see figure 8.7).

Explore different arm positions—alongside your body, out to the sides, or stretched in front of you—to continue challenging your balance.

Play with your balance for a few breaths, then bring your leg back down and return to Mountain pose.

Repeat on the other side.

When you are done, stand in Mountain pose and notice the various responses—in your body and mind—that rise in response to balance challenges.

Remember

- Keep your breath flowing.

- Keep softness in the knee of your supporting leg.

- Notice if there is any difference between your ability to balance on the right or left leg.

Caution

- If you are tall and have to stoop over to rest your fingers on the chair, practice with a wall as your support.

Eagle

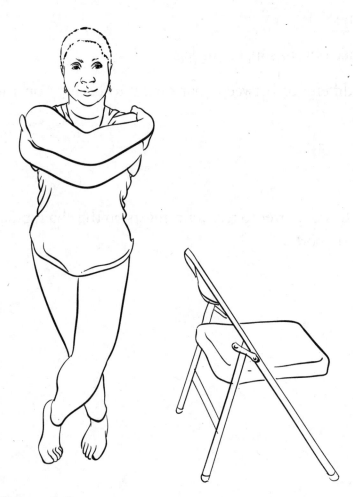

Figure 8.8

Setup

Stand behind or beside your chair close enough to lightly hold on to the back of the chair for support. Position your feet hip-width apart, and feel the ground beneath your feet.

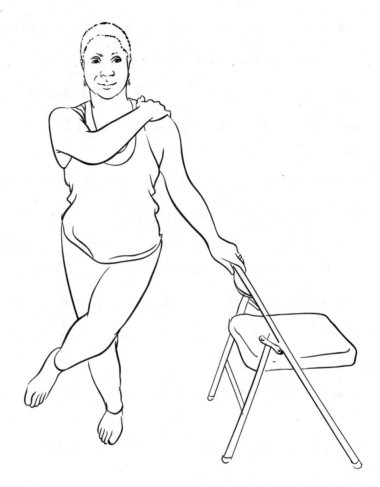

Figure 8.9

Movement

Stand tall in Mountain pose.

Inhale your arms out to the sides of your body so that they are extended at shoulder height.

Exhale and cross your right arm over your left arm in front of your chest, as close to your chest as is comfortable.

Land the right hand on the left shoulder and the left hand on the right shoulder.

Keep your shoulders relaxed as you invite your elbows to lift off of your chest.

Focus your gaze at a point on the horizon.

Shift the weight of your body into your right leg, keeping your hips steady.

Take a baby step forward with your left foot as you send "roots" down your right leg.

If this feels steady, move your left foot in front of your right foot.

If you still feel balanced, step your left foot over your right foot (see figure 8.8).

If this feels steady, lift your left foot off the ground, hugging your thighs together. Feel free to touch the chair for support with one hand if you like (see figure 8.9).

Find the position that allows you to maintain your balance.

Take a few easy breaths in the position where you feel challenged but comfortable.

Inhale and step your feet back into Mountain pose, extending your arms out to the side.

Exhale and relax your arms down to your sides.

Repeat on the other side.

When you are done, stand in Mountain pose and breathe comfortably.

Remember

- Check in with your balance at each step. Be sure you feel steady before you progress further.

- Notice any differences in how the standing leg feels after the pose.

- Feel the responses of the body: the sensations, the emotions, the thoughts, the breath.

- Pay attention to any self-talk, and remember to treat yourself with kindness.

- Stay present with the experience of the body letting go of the posture.

Tight Rope

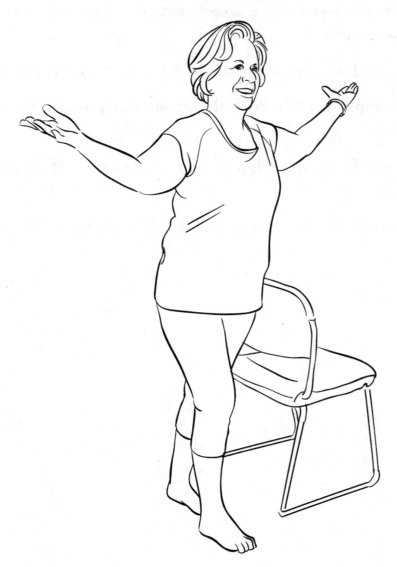

Figure 8.10 Tight Rope pose

Setup

Stand beside your chair close enough to lightly hold on to the back of the chair for support. Position your feet hip-width apart, and feel the ground beneath your feet.

Movement

Stand tall in Mountain pose.

Inhale your arms out to the sides of your body so that they are extended at about shoulder height.

Exhale and soften your shoulders, your elbows, and your hands.

Focus your gaze at a point on the horizon.

Shift the weight of your body into your left leg, keeping your hips steady.

Take a baby step forward with your right foot and check in to see how balanced you are.

If this feels steady, move your right foot toward your left foot.

If you still feel balanced, step your right heel directly in front of your left foot, as if you are walking on a tight rope (see figure 8.10).

Shift your weight forward into your right foot, lifting your left heel.

Shift your weight back into your left foot.

Practice slowly shifting your weight from your front foot to your back foot.

For further challenge, explore stepping your right foot behind your left foot.

Continue practicing this weight shifting, keeping your breath flowing comfortably.

When you're ready, step back into Mountain pose.

Then repeat this sequence by stepping the left foot forward first.

When you're done, step back into Mountain pose and breathe comfortably.

Remember

- Check in with your balance at each step before you progress to the next step.

- Always feel free to rest when necessary.

- Notice all of the small changes inherent in balance.

Caution

- If balancing with one foot in front of the other is too challenging, widen your stance as if you were "walking a plank" rather than a tightrope.

CHAPTER 9

Week 5: Back Strengthening to Support Healthy Posture

Finding ways to keep your back strong as you age is important. Metaphorically, having a strong back allows us to be in the world with a sense of dignity and elegance. Physically, having a weak back contributes to back pain and a corresponding decreased ability to engage in meaningful activities. In fact, back pain is one of our society's most common medical problems.[110] The practices introduced in this chapter are designed to strengthen your back so you can enjoy healthy posture, decreased pain, and fuller participation in life.

> Having a strong back allows us to be in the world with a sense of dignity and elegance.

Functional Benefits of the Back-Strengthening Practice

Strengthens weak muscles. Practicing sustained backbends can recondition the muscles of the back body that tend to get weak with disuse.

Enables prolonged activities. Having a strong back can make it more comfortable to sit through a grandchild's soccer game or the symphony, stargaze, or take a nice stroll through your favorite park.

Counters the tendency to slump. Back-strengthening postures also stretch and lengthen the front of the body, countering the tendency to slump forward and creating more space for the organs of respiration, circulation, and digestion.

As a reminder, you can download audio for week 5's practice at http://www.newharbinger.com/33643.

Supple Spine Flow

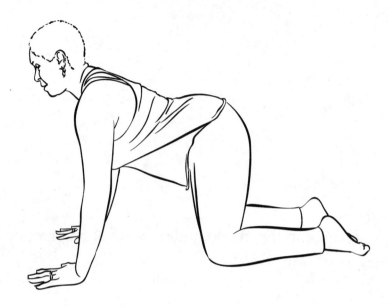

Figure 9.1

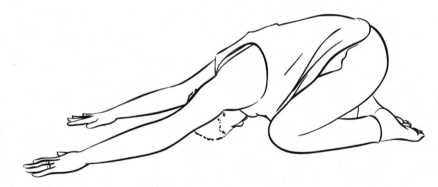

Figure 9.2

Setup

Come down onto your hands and knees on a mat or soft carpet. In this table-top position, place your hands under your shoulders and your knees under your hips. Feel free to cushion your wrists and/or your knees with a folded towel or other prop.

Movement

Inhale as you lift and extend your breastbone toward the wall in front of you and your tailbone toward the wall behind you (see figure 9.1).

Exhale as you drop your tailbone down and relax your head toward the ground. Avoid emphasizing the rounding of your upper back as you relax your head and tailbone down—in other words, do not press down with your arms to strongly round your back.

Inhale and lift your heart forward and your tailbone up and back—so your spine arches in two directions, like a smile.

Exhale and relax your tailbone and your head down.

Continue extending and articulating your spine in this way for a few breaths, trying to synchronize your movement with your breath.

Next, as you exhale and drop your tailbone and head, also move your buttocks as close as they will come to your heels (see figure 9.2). This posture is known as Child's pose.

Inhale back to hands and knees, and extend your heart forward and your tailbone behind you.

Exhale as you drop your tailbone and move your buttocks back toward your heels again into Child's pose.

Continue this rhythm for a few breaths.

Then pause with your buttocks as close to your heels as they will comfortably go, and relax your head toward the ground. If your forehead doesn't comfortably reach the ground, please give it a place to rest—be sure your head doesn't just hang. You might stack your palms or fists and rest your forehead on them. Or, if you prefer, rest your forehead on a block or cushion.

Relax here for several breaths, inviting your breath to nourish your low back, waist, shoulder blades, and neck.

Remember

- If your wrists aren't able to support the weight of the arms and shoulders, explore coming onto your fists or lowering down onto your forearms.

- If your knees and/or wrists are sensitive, try placing a pillow or a rolled towel under them.

- Bring your buttocks back toward your heels only as far as is comfortable.

- Welcome the simple pleasure of just being.

Caution

- Avoid pressing into the ground with your hands when your head and tail-bone are dropped. Pushing your spine into this rounded "Halloween cat" position can place too much force on the vertebrae.

Crocodile

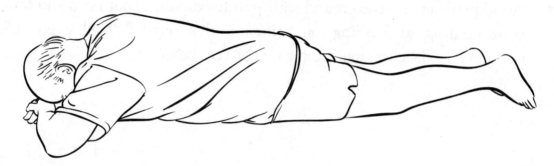

Figure 9.3 Crocodile pose

Setup

Come down to rest on your belly. Bend your elbows and stack your hands to make a little pillow for your head, turning your neck so that your cheek or your ear rests on the back of your hands. If it's uncomfortable to turn your head in this position, please rest your forehead or chin on the back of your hands (see figure 9.3).

Movement

Allow your body to relax completely, so your weight releases down into the earth.

Let your heels turn away from each other.

Take a few slow, deep breaths.

Feel your back body expand with the inhalation and relax on the exhalation.

If you are resting on your cheek or ear, turn your head to the other side for a few breaths.

Remember

- Notice the effects of this gravitational and energetic shift.

- Completely surrender your body weight into the earth.

- Be aware of the sensations in your physical body, any waves of emotion, and any thoughts in your thinking mind.

- If lying on your belly is uncomfortable for your feet or legs, try putting a rolled towel under your ankles.

Sphinx

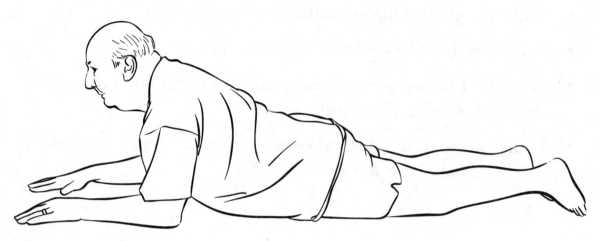

Figure 9.4 Sphinx pose

Setup

Rest on your belly. Place your elbows under your shoulders and bring your forearms parallel to each other with your palms on the ground.

Movement

Root the front of your pelvis into the ground.

Lengthen your legs behind you and press the tops of your feet into the ground (see figure 9.4).

Draw your shoulders back and down.

Beginning with your tailbone, invite each vertebra to extend forward and up.

Lengthen up through the crown of your head.

Continue to lengthen back through your legs.

Root your forearms into the ground as you explore the action of "pulling the ground toward you" isometrically.

Breathe into your belly and chest for several breaths.

When you are ready to come out of this backbend, open your elbows out to the sides and pull the ground toward you with your hands to lengthen the spine.

Rest on the ground for several breaths. Then return to Crocodile pose one more time, if you like.

Remember

- Feel how and where the breath moves after a backbend.

- Notice if you feel a sensation of stretching across the front of your torso.

Baby Cobra

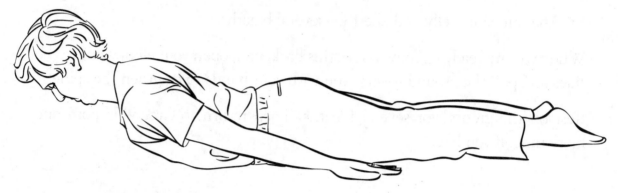

Figure 9.5 Baby Cobra pose

Setup

Rest on your belly with your elbows bent, one hand placed on top of the other as in Crocodile pose. Rest your cheek, chin, or forehead on the back of your stacked hands. Pause here and take several belly-focused breaths.

Movement

Move your arms down along your sides, palms down. Rest your forehead or chin on the ground.

Root the front of your pelvis into the ground.

Extend your legs back and press the tops of your feet into the ground.

Shrug your shoulders back and down.

Inhale and lift your head, shoulders, and chest up off the ground (see figure 9.5).

Exhale and soften a bit so that your body moves slightly back toward the ground.

Continue with this integration of breath and posture: inhale and lift, exhale and soften.

Keep energy moving down through your legs.

Explore remaining in the lifted position while still feeling the rise and fall of the breath.

On an exhalation, release back to the ground and rest.

Breathe into your back and notice where your breath moves.

Remember

- Only lift your head, shoulders, and chest as high as comfortable. Your strength will build over time with practice.

- Keep the front and back of your neck long, without jutting the chin forward. This means your gaze will likely be down, not forward.

Locust

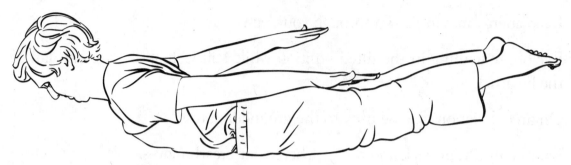

Figure 9.6 Locust pose

Setup

Lie on your belly with your elbows bent and your cheek, chin, or forehead resting on your stacked palms. Pause here and take a few belly-focused breaths.

Movement

Move your arms down along your sides, palms down. Rest your forehead on the ground.

Root the front of your pelvis into the ground.

Extend your legs back and press the tops of your feet into the ground.

Draw your shoulders back and down.

Inhale and lift your head, shoulders, chest, arms, and legs away from the ground (see figure 9.6).

Exhale and soften a bit, so your body moves slightly back toward the ground.

Continue with this integration of breath and posture: inhale and lift, exhale and soften.

Balance the amount of energy in the upper body with the amount in the lower body.

Explore remaining in the lifted position while still feeling the rise and fall of the breath.

On an exhalation, release back to the ground and rest.

Breathe into the back and notice where the breath moves.

Remember

- Only lift your head, shoulders, chest, arms, and legs as high as comfortable. Your strength will build over time with practice.

- Keep the front and back of the neck long, without jutting the chin forward. This means your gaze will likely be down, not forward.

- When you finish the posture and rest, keep your attention present with the experience of your body letting go. Pay attention to how this feels.

Bridge

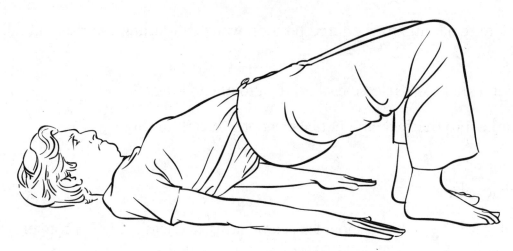

Figure 9.7 Bridge pose

Setup

Lie on your back with your knees bent. Place your feet flat on the ground and hip-width apart. Rest your arms at your sides, palms down. Tune in to your breath.

Movement

Inhale and root down with your feet and arms as you lift your hips up off the ground (see figure 9.7).

Exhale and release your hips back down.

Continue with this easy lifting and lowering: inhale your hips up and exhale them down. Try to keep your legs parallel—avoid letting your knees "knock" in or splay out.

For more challenge, stay in the "up" position for a few slow, full breaths.

When you are done, return your hips to the ground and rest.

Remember

- Be sure your head is properly aligned: your chin should be in line with the little "notch" in your collarbones.

- Bring your chin slightly lower than your forehead, but don't flatten your neck. Be sure to keep the natural curve in your neck so that there is a little space behind it.

- Keep your breath flowing. Avoid holding your breath.

- Only lift your hips as high as comfortable. Your strength will build over time with practice.

Knees to Chest

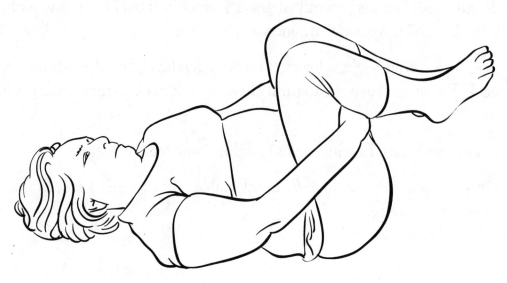

Figure 9.8 Knees-to-Chest pose

Setup

Lie on your back with your knees bent, feet flat on the ground, and arms at your sides. If your chin is higher than your forehead, place a folded blanket or towel behind your head so that your chin is at the same level—or slightly below—your forehead. Tune in to your breath.

Movement

Bring both knees toward your chest as close as is comfortable.

Hold on to your legs behind your knees or on top of your shins (see figure 9.8).

Welcome breath into the back of your body—your tailbone, your love handles, behind your heart.

Linger here for several breaths. You might notice that, as you inhale and fill your body with breath, your thighs move slightly away from your body. As you exhale and release used air, you might hug your thighs in just a little more and feel the sensation of stretch in your low back.

After 3 to 5 breaths, or when you are ready, return the soles of the feet to the ground with your knees bent.

Remember

- If it feels like a strain to hold your legs with your hands, use a strap over your shins or behind your thighs to keep your thighs close to your belly. If this still feels stressful, let your arms rest at your sides. You can also hug one leg at a time if that is more comfortable. If you have knee arthritis, it may be more comfortable to hold behind your thighs instead of holding your shins.

- Feel free to widen your thighs to make room for your belly, if you like.

- Notice how the waves of breath and the waves of sensation come into relationship.

- Discover the various responses—physical, emotional, mental, energetic—to the posture.

CHAPTER 10

Week 6: Core Strengthening to Enhance Spinal Health

Discovering strength in our center, in our core, is desirable for various reasons. Metaphorically, feeling strong and steady in our center helps us stay focused and connected to our inner resources. Physically, feeling strong in our core helps maintain spinal and functional health. Balanced core strength includes more than sit-ups, which tend to mostly strengthen the superficial abdominal muscles. True core strength focuses on the deeper layers of abdominal muscles in the front of the belly and the sides of the torso, as well as the muscles that support the spine and pelvis. The practices introduced in this chapter are designed to help you build strength in your core to enliven your center.

> Practicing the art of welcoming whatever arises, even if it's something difficult—such as a physical or emotional pain—can be essential to finding freedom from suffering.

Functional Benefits of the Core-Strengthening Practice

Relieves back pain. A strong core provides a healthy foundation for all the body's movements and is a key component in relieving back pain.

Builds strength required for daily activities. Maintaining core strength allows us to continue participating in many of our daily activities, such as tying our shoes, dressing, housecleaning, and cooking.

Expands the potential for recreation. Many of our recreational pleasures—golfing, gardening, tennis, and physical intimacy—are all supported by good core strength.

As a reminder, you can download audio for week 6's practice at http://
www.newharbinger.com/33643.

Royal Cough

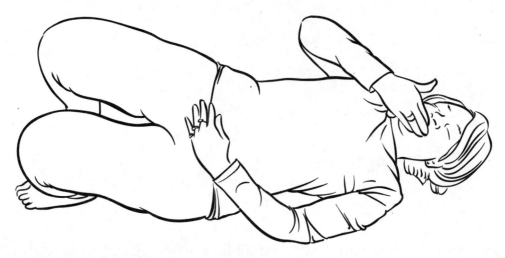

Figure 10.1 Royal Cough pose

Setup

Lie on your back with your knees bent, feet flat on the ground, and arms at your sides. If your chin is higher than your forehead, place a folded blanket or towel behind your head so that your chin is at the same level or slightly below your forehead. Tune in to your breath.

Movement

Place one hand on your lower belly and the other over your mouth, then cough (see figure 10.1).

Notice how your abdominal muscles engage and your belly bounces when you cough.

Now, practice engaging the muscles that are activated when you cough, but without actually coughing. Explore this action without interfering with your breath.

Next, relax your abdominals completely as you inhale, feeling your belly round, just as you do in Three-Part Breath.

This time, as you exhale, engage your abdominals and draw your belly in toward your spine. Practice this pattern several times: relaxed abdominal muscles on an inhalation, engaged abdominal muscles on an exhalation.

Remember

- Notice how your body feels when your abdominals are engaged and when they are not.

- Try to draw in your abdominal muscles without compromising your breath.

One-Legged Bicycle

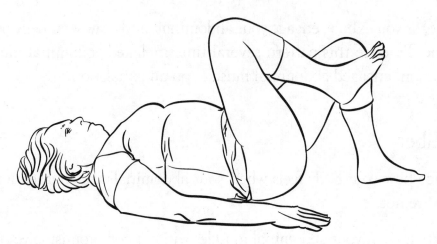

Figure 10.2

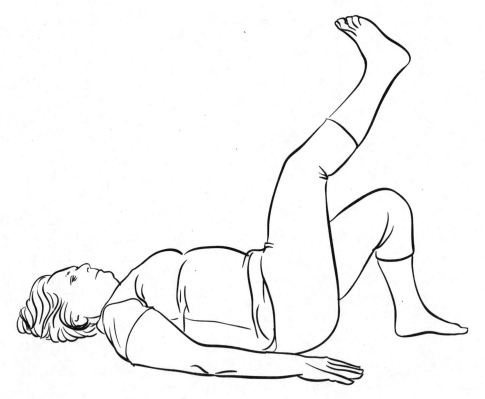

Figure 10.3

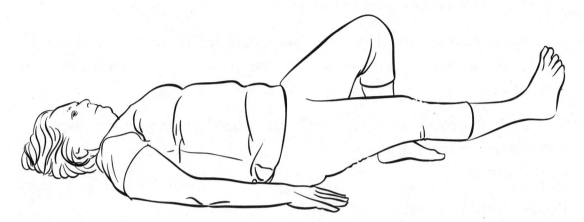

Figure 10.4

Setup

Lie on your back with your knees bent, feet flat on the ground and hip-width apart. Position your head so that your neck maintains its natural curve. Place your arms along your sides, palms down. Tune in to your breath.

Movement

Lift your right foot off the ground and bring your right knee in toward your belly (see figure 10.2).

Inhale and extend your right leg up toward the sky, flexing your ankle (see figure 10.3).

Exhale and engage the deep belly muscles of the Royal Cough (see page 168) as you lower your leg until it is just above the ground (see figure 10.4).

Inhale and bend your right knee, bringing it back in toward your belly, then extend your right leg back up toward the sky.

Exhale and lower your leg until it is just above the ground, engaging the strength in your center.

Repeat a couple of times at your own pace.

To build more strength, linger with your right leg hovering just above the ground for a couple of breaths. Be sure to keep your breath flowing comfortably.

When you are ready, exhale your leg to the ground and notice the cascade of release when gravity takes over and your leg can rest. Pause here to be present for this letting go.

Repeat on the other side.

When you are done, place both feet on the ground, knees bent, and enjoy several smooth breaths.

Remember

- Engage only the muscles that you need, softening what you don't need. Be sure to keep your upper body—shoulders, neck, and face—relaxed.

- Find ease in your breath. If you need more than one breath to extend your leg or bend your knee, that's fine. Just do your best and avoid holding your breath.

Caution

- Be sure to bend your knee toward your belly before extending your leg straight up. Avoid lifting a straight leg up from the ground.

- If your low back feels strained, try rooting your low back into the ground by engaging your belly throughout the movement.

Lake Mudra

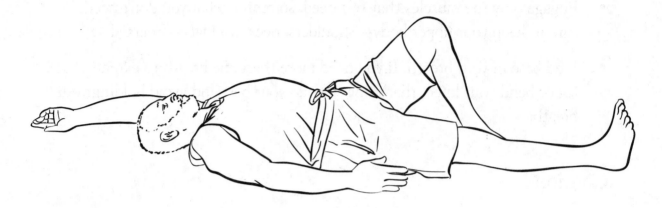

Figure 10.5 Lake Mudra pose

Setup

Lie on your back with your knees bent, feet flat on the ground about hip-width apart. Extend your arms down by your sides with your palms facing your thighs. Tune in to your breath.

Movement

Inhale and extend your left arm up and back toward your ear as you extend your right leg out, hovering a few inches above the ground (see figure 10.5).

Exhale and return your arm and leg to the starting position.

Inhale and extend your right arm and left leg, lengthening across the diagonal.

Exhale and return to the starting position.

Continue with this movement, inhaling to extend your opposite limbs across the diagonal and exhaling to return to the starting position.

Engage your lower belly, drawing it in toward your spine to stabilize your pelvis.

For more challenge, explore pausing in the extended position. Keep your breath fluid. Practice engaging the strength in your center.

Play with this practice for several breaths, challenging your core. When you are ready to rest, bring your arms back along your sides, bend your knees, and bring the soles of your feet to the ground. Pause here and notice how you feel.

Remember

- If your low back feels strained, emphasize drawing your lower belly strongly to the spine and rooting your low back into the ground throughout the movement. You may also slide your leg out along the ground, letting it touch down instead of hovering above the ground.

- Remain curious as to how your body, mind, and heart are responding to the experience.

Spinal Balance

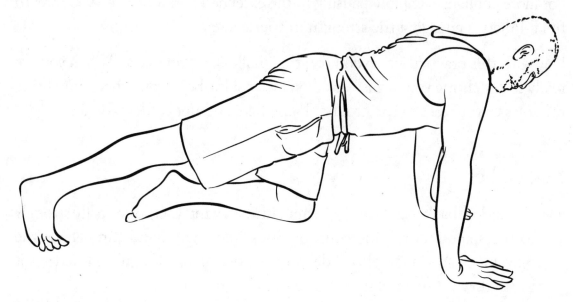

Figure 10.6

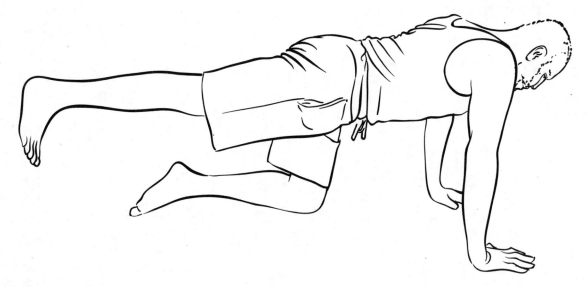

Figure 10.7

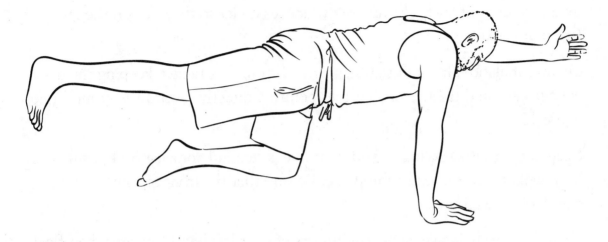

Figure 10.8

Setup

Come onto your hands and knees on a mat or soft carpet. In this tabletop position, place your hands under your shoulders and your knees under your hips. Feel free to cushion your wrists and/or your knees with a folded towel or other prop. Tune in to your breath.

Movement

Root down into your hands. Feel a sense of aliveness in your arms and chest. Be sure to keep length in your spine, with the top of your head extending forward and your tailbone extending back.

Draw your belly toward your spine using the action of the Royal Cough (see page 168).

Extend your right leg back and tuck your toes under so they rest on the ground (see figure 10.6).

On an inhalation, lift your right leg up with your foot flexed, keeping the front of your knee and the tips of your toes pointing directly toward the ground (see figure 10.7).

Keep your breath flowing as you continue to extend your leg back, as if your heel could touch the wall behind you. Be sure that the front of your right hip is parallel to the ground.

To add more challenge, crawl the fingers of your left hand forward, then float your left arm up (see figure 10.8).

Rotate the palm of your left hand so that your thumb is pointing toward the sky.

Maintain strength and awareness in your belly to support your extended limbs by hugging the belly to the spine.

Lengthen across the diagonal of your body, extending from the fingertips of your left hand to the heel of your right foot.

After a few breaths, return your hand and knee to the ground.

Relax your head and let your tailbone be heavy.

Breathe into your back.

Repeat on the other side.

When you are finished, feel free to rest for several breaths in Child's pose.

Remember

- Let your breath be easy.

- If your knees are uncomfortable, try placing a pillow or rolled towel under them.

- If this position is too demanding for your wrists, try coming down onto your forearms, or make fists and balance on your knuckles. Sometimes a little cushion under the heels of your hands (such as a folded washcloth) can help.

Caution

- Avoid pushing into your hands too strongly—be sure not to round your back when you root down into your hands.

Plank Progression

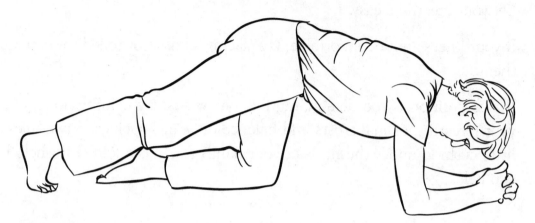

Figure 10.9

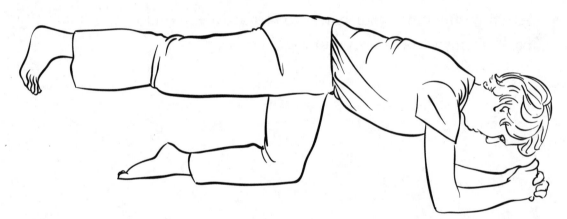

Figure 10.10

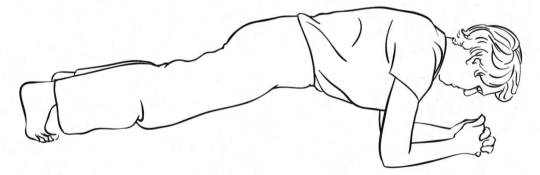

Figure 10.11

Setup

Come onto your hands and knees on a mat or soft carpet. Lower your forearms to the ground, with your elbows under your shoulders. Interlace your fingers and create a tripod of support. Tune in to your breath.

Movement

Engage the muscles of your lower belly using the action of the Royal Cough (see page 168).

Draw your shoulders back and down.

Root your forearms into the ground to engage your arms and chest.

Step your right leg back, toes tucked under so they rest on the mat or carpet (see figure 10.9).

Balance your weight between your right and left arms.

Explore lifting your right leg up to the height of your hip, toes and knee facing down (see figure 10.10).

Take a few easy breaths, then return your right knee to the ground.

Step your left leg back, toes tucked under, and balance the weight evenly between both arms.

Explore lifting your left leg up to the height of your hip, toes and knee facing down.

Breathe here until you are ready to return your left knee to the ground.

To increase the challenge, explore stepping both legs back with the toes tucked under (see figure 10.11).

Extend your tailbone toward your heels, root into the ground with your forearms, and engage the muscles of your belly.

Maintain ease in your breath.

When you are done, release your knees to the ground and stretch your back by bringing your hips toward your heels in Child's pose.

Remember

- Keep your breath flowing smoothly.

- Move through the variations as you feel ready. There is no rush. Strength will build over time.

CHAPTER 11

Additional Practices to Enhance Vigor and Relaxation

Now that you've spent six weeks learning to Relax into Yoga, you might enjoy trying the following sequences for more challenge and variety. You can repeat one of these flowing sequences multiple times to build endurance and invigorate your body. Although both the flowing sequences as well as the relaxation sequence could be done as a stand-alone, focused practice, we recommend warming up with the practices from week 1 (Three-Part Breath and Range-of-Motion Sequence) and finishing with Relaxation pose.

As a reminder, you can download audio for these additional practices at http://www.newharbinger.com/33643.

Flowing Sequences to Build Endurance and Enhance Vigor

Functional Benefits of the Flowing Sequences

- **Build strength and endurance.** These flowing sequences of standing postures require continued use of the large muscles of the body, which—over time—can enhance your strength and stamina.

- **Boost balance.** The rhythmic movements in these sequences, particularly those asking you to step from two legs to one, can enhance your ability to keep your body upright.

- **Offer brain training.** The choreography of the flowing sequences challenges the brain to learn how to link postures together. Just like learning to dance, it can be great fun.

> **Please recognize that yoga is not just about training your body—you are also training your mind.**

Sun Salutation at the Wall

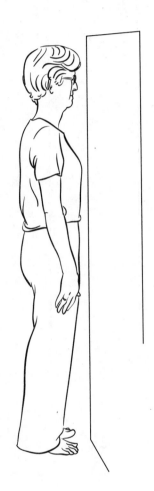

Figure 11.1

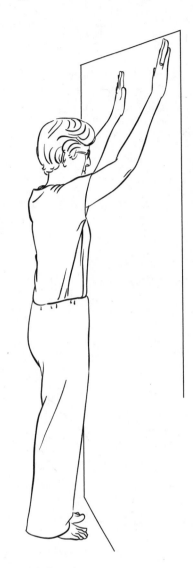

Figure 11.2

Setup

Stand tall facing a wall in Mountain pose, with your toes several inches from the wall (see figure 11.1). Feel the four corners of your feet anchor firmly into the ground. Slightly drop your tailbone, engage your belly, and lift your heart. Feel your breath.

Movement

Sweep your arms out to the sides and over your head, landing your palms on the wall shoulder-width apart or as wide as is comfortable (see figure 11.2).

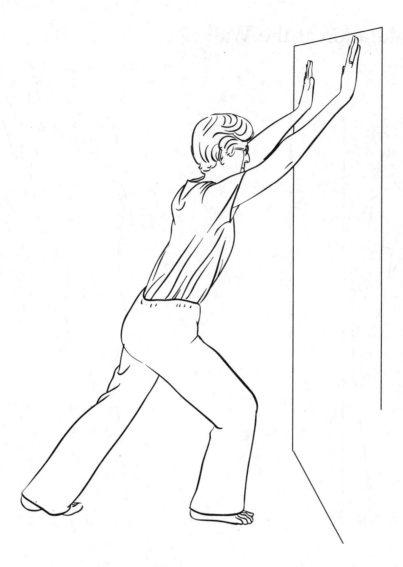

Figure 11.3

Step your left leg back behind you as far as is comfortable, placing the ball of your foot on the ground and keeping the heel lifted.

Bend your right knee, making sure that it does not bend so far forward that you can't see your toes (see figure 11.3).

Step your left foot forward a couple of inches.

Step your right foot back beside your left.

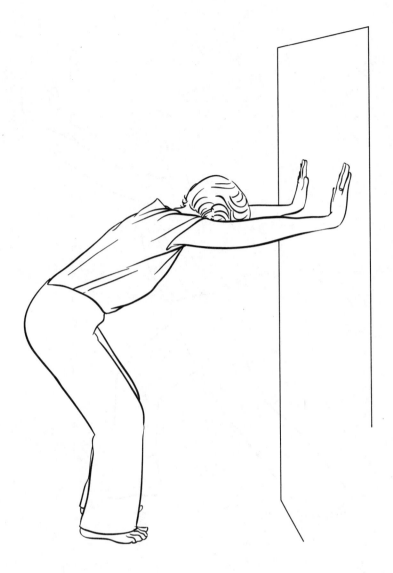

Figure 11.4

Bend your knees and extend your tailbone to the wall behind you, sliding your hands down the wall (keeping them shoulder-width apart) so you can lengthen your spine (see figure 11.4).

Step your left foot forward toward the wall and slide your right foot back a few inches.

Bend your left knee so it is over your ankle and aligned with your toes.

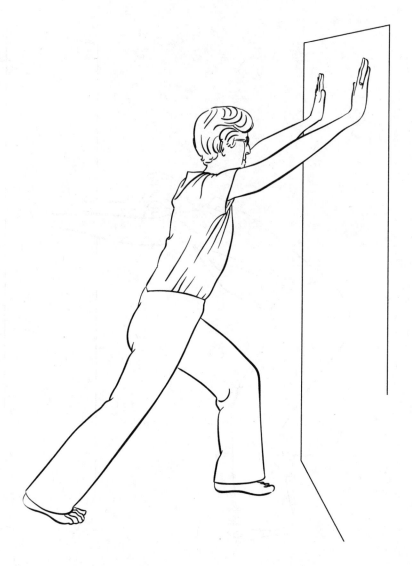

Figure 11.5

Slide your arms back up the wall, still shoulder-width apart (see figure 11.5).

Step your right foot forward by the left and slide your hands down the wall until they are in front of your ribs (see figure 11.6).

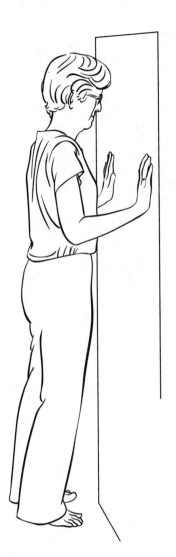 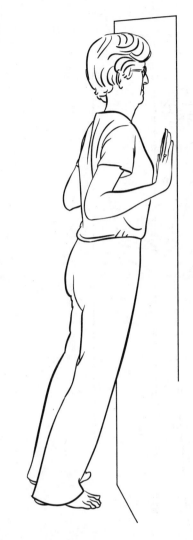

Figure 11.6   **Figure 11.7**

Engage your belly and hug your elbows toward your body. Invite your shoulders back and down, and tilt your tailbone toward the ground.

Bend your elbows to "lower" your straight body toward the wall, as if lowering into a push-up (see figure 11.7).

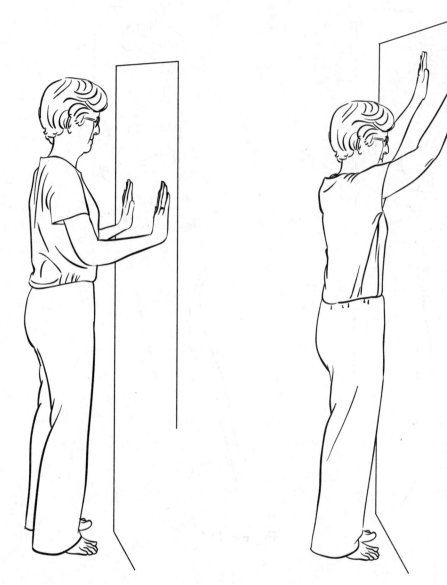

Figure 11.8   **Figure 11.9**

Press the wall away with your hands (see figure 11.8) and slide your palms back up the wall as high as is comfortable (see figure 11.9).

Sweep your arms out and down and return to Mountain pose (see figure 11.10).

Feel free to continue for several more cycles of Sun Salutation at the Wall.

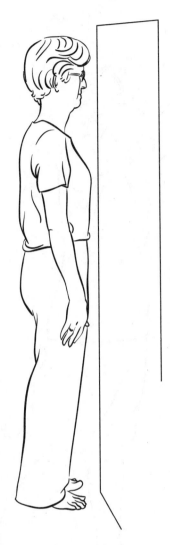

Figure 11.10

Remember

- Keep your bent knee over your ankle and aligned with your second toe to avoid straining your knee.

- Practice keeping your spine long when you extend your tailbone to the back wall. If you feel your spine curving in this position, bend your knees more deeply.

- Pause between rounds and take an easy breath. Feel the ground below you and the sky above you. Find the strength of a mountain.

- Become aware of the various responses of your body, mind, and heart to this sequence.

Caution

- Avoid bending your knee so deeply that it goes beyond your toes. If you can't see your toes when you look down, bend your knee less.

- Avoid pushing your back heel to the ground. Rather, let the heel stay lifted.

Crane to Crescent

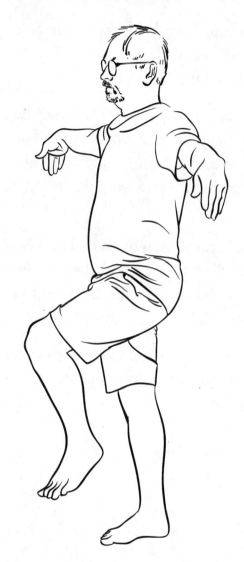

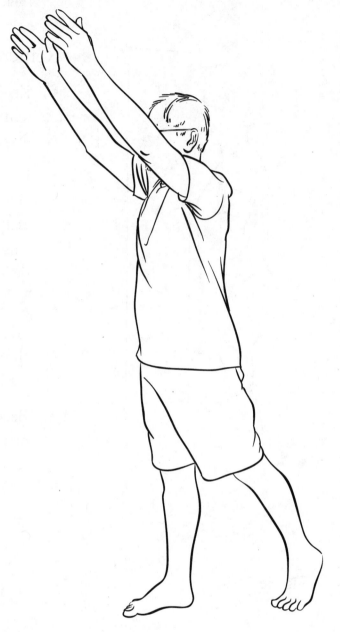

Figure 11.11

Figure 11.12

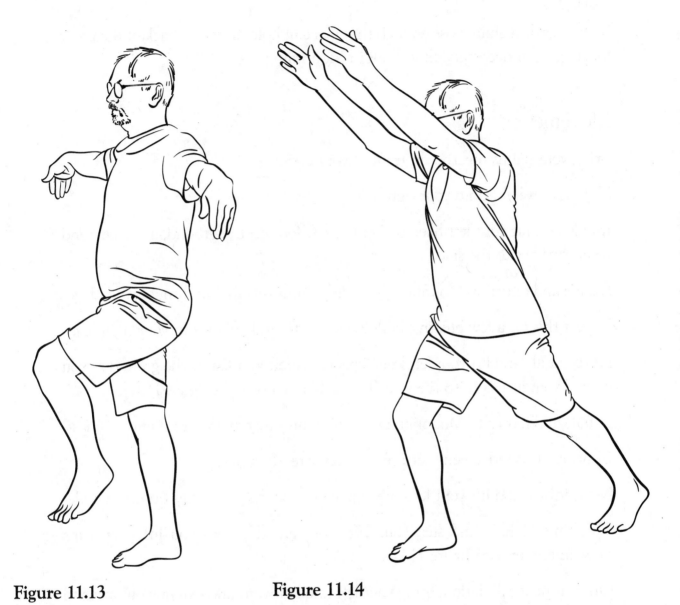

Figure 11.13

Figure 11.14

Setup

Stand beside a chair close enough that you can hold on to the back of the chair for support, if necessary. Stand tall in Mountain pose.

Movement

Bring your palms together in front of your chest.

Shift your weight onto your right leg.

Inhale and lift your left heel, ball of the left foot on the ground, as you extend your arms out to the side.

Exhale and return to Mountain pose with palms together in front of your chest.

Repeat this for a few breaths, building strength and balance in your right leg.

Next, inhale and lift your left knee up so your left foot leaves the ground as you extend your arms out to the side. This is Crane pose (see figure 11.11).

Exhale and return to Mountain pose with palms together in front of your chest.

Continue this movement pattern for a few breath cycles.

Next, inhale and lift your left knee up as you extend your arms out to the side.

This time, exhale and step your left foot behind you as you lift your arms forward and up (see figure 11.12).

On your next inhalation, bring your left knee forward and extend your arms to the sides in Crane pose (see figure 11.13).

Exhale and return to Mountain pose with palms together in front of your chest.

Continue for several breaths.

For more challenge, step your left foot a bit farther behind you and bend your right knee as your sweep your arms forward and up. This is Crescent pose (see figure 11.14).

Inhale and bring your left knee forward and your arms out to the side in Crane pose.

Exhale and return to Mountain pose with palms together in front of your chest. Pause for a few breaths, simply breathing.

Repeat on the other side: stand on your left leg and move your right leg.

Remember

- Feel free to add the breath pattern after you become familiar with the sequence.

- Explore the variation that is challenging but does not cause strain.

- Use the chair for support if your balance is unsteady.

- Keep your breath fluid.

Chair Flow

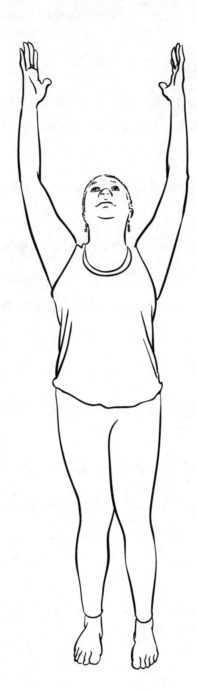

Figure 11.15

Setup

Stand tall in Mountain pose.

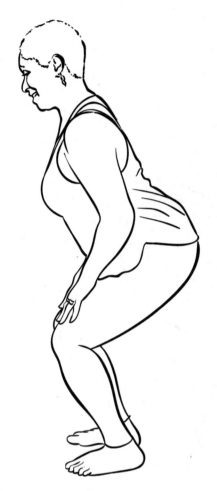

Figure 11.16

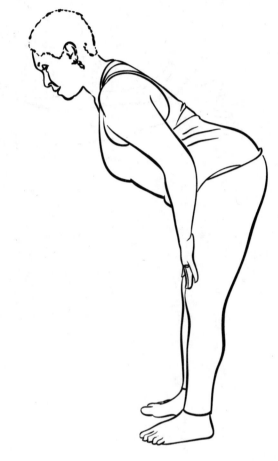

Figure 11.17

Movement

Inhale and sweep your arms out and up (see figure 11.15).

Exhale and hinge forward from your hips as you bend your knees and extend your bottom back into Chair pose, bringing your hands to your thighs (see figure 11.16).

Inhale and press your palms into your thighs as you straighten your legs and lengthen your back (see figure 11.17).

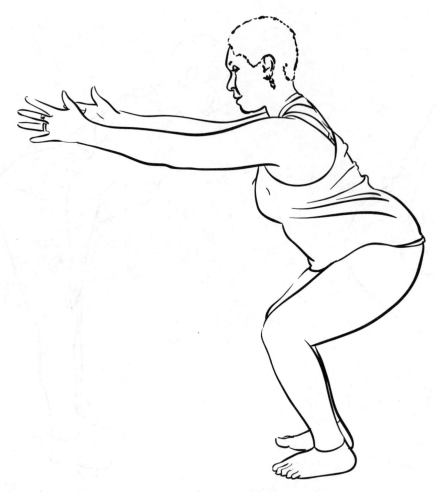

Figure 11.18

Exhale and float your arms forward as you bend your knees and draw your bottom back into Chair pose (see figure 11.18).

Inhale and root into your feet, straighten your legs, and extend your arms out and up, gazing up and coming to standing (see figure 11.19).

Exhale and sweep your arms out to the sides and come back to Mountain pose (see figure 11.20).

Continue for several cycles, or as long as it feels nourishing.

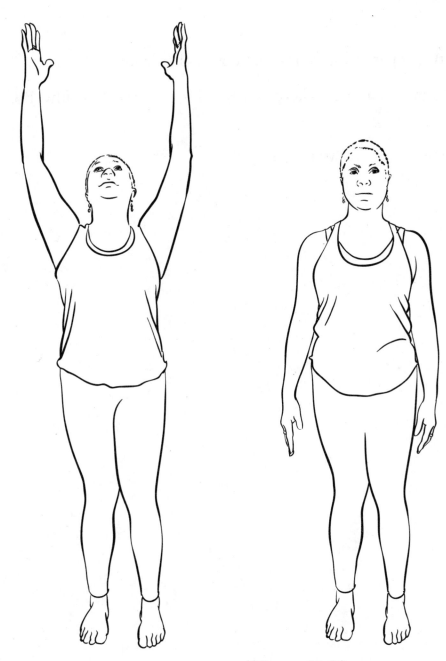

Figure 11.19   **Figure 11.20**

When you are finished, rest your palms on your chest for a few moments and feel the effect this practice has on your breath, your heart, your body, and your mind.

Remember

- Keep your thighs parallel so your knees don't collapse into each other.

- Avoid rounding your back—keep a neutral spine (see "Healthy Body Mechanics," page 52).

- Feel free to rest whenever you need to.

Quieting Practices to Stretch and Relax

Functional Benefits of the Quieting Practices

- **Ease tension.** Deep, relaxed stretching can help release tension from body and mind.

- **Enhance flexibility.** Stretching tight muscles can improve joint mobility.

- **Relieve pain.** Relaxing in the presence of stretching sensations can help the brain and central nervous system learn a different response to the sensations of persistent pain.

- **Calm the nervous system.** Quieting practices can trigger the relaxation response, which involves a cascade of calming physiologic changes, including decreased heart rate, blood pressure, and breathing rate.

- **Connect to quieter dimensions of experience.** The stillness that can arise with the quieting practices can be a deeply welcome place of rest for body, mind, heart, and spirit.

> Relax into Yoga cultivates the critical counterbalance of undoing, of slowing down, of savoring the moment and knowing more fully what life is presenting *right now.*

Hand to Big Toe

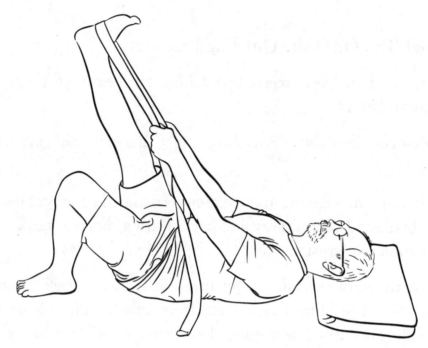

Figure 11.21

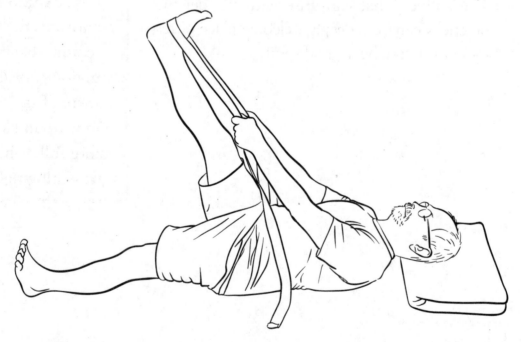

Figure 11.22

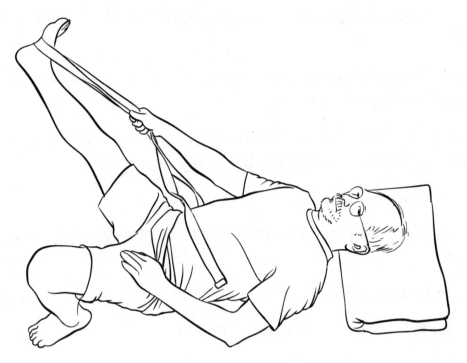

Figure 11.23

Setup

Rest on your back with your knees bent and the soles of your feet flat on the ground. Have a strap nearby. Bring your arms alongside your body, palms down, and tune in to your breath.

Movement

Bend your right knee toward your belly and place a strap around the ball or arch of your right foot.

Inhale and extend your right foot up toward the sky, straightening your leg as much as you comfortably can. Keep your left knee bent, with your left foot on the ground (see figure 11.21).

Exhale and flex your right foot as you let your right thigh be heavy in the hip socket.

Pause here for several breaths, extending up through your right heel and releasing down through your right hip.

To deepen the stretch, extend your left leg along the ground, flexing your left foot and pointing your toes toward the sky (see figure 11.22).

Take several breaths here.

Take both sides of the strap in your right hand and place your left hand on your left thigh.

Bend your left knee again so that the sole of your left foot is flat on the ground.

Open your right leg to the right (see figure 11.23).

Keep your left hip and buttock heavy on the ground and allow your left knee to drift slightly to the left to help you counterbalance the weight of your extended right leg. Place your left hand on your left thigh or hip to keep the left side of your pelvis from lifting up.

Linger here for several breaths.

Inhale and bring your right leg back to center.

Exhale and allow your right foot to return to the ground.

Repeat on the other side.

Remember

- Extend the lifted leg only as long as is comfortable.

- If your chin juts upward and the back of your neck feels crunched, place a folded towel under your head.

- If you are unable (or prefer not) to get down on the ground, try this practice lying in your bed.

- Keep your shoulders relaxed and on the ground. You may need to slide your hands down the strap to avoid creating stress in your hands, arms, and shoulders.

- As you lengthen into the stretch, bring attention to the different qualities of sensation that are present.

Supine Bound Angle

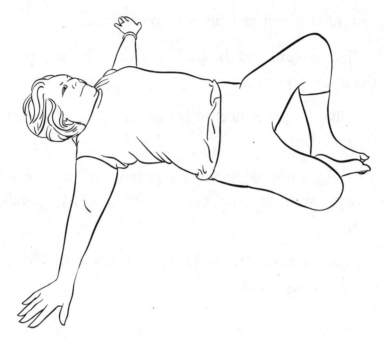

Figure 11.24

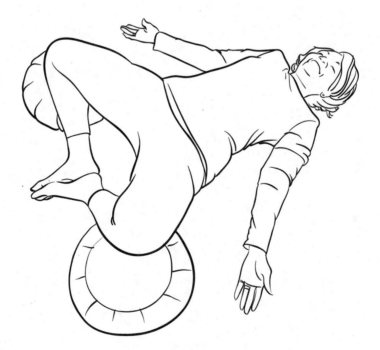

Figure 11.25

Setup

Rest on your back with your knees bent and the soles of your feet flat on the ground. You may want to have a couple of pillows nearby.

Movement

Bring the soles of your feet together and let your knees open out to the sides.

Extend your arms out to the sides (see figure 11.24). Your palms can be up or down, whichever feels best to you.

Breathe into your hips and groin. If you are unable to relax in this position, tuck a pillow under each thigh for support (see figure 11.25).

Linger here for several breaths, inviting your legs and hips to relax and release.

When you are ready to come out of the pose, place your hands on your outer thighs and use the strength of your hands and arms to help return your thighs to the starting position.

Remember

- Try this pose with and without a support under your thighs to see which variation invites greater relaxation.

- Feel free to cover yourself with a blanket for comfort if you'd like to rest in this position for a little while.

Legs on a Chair

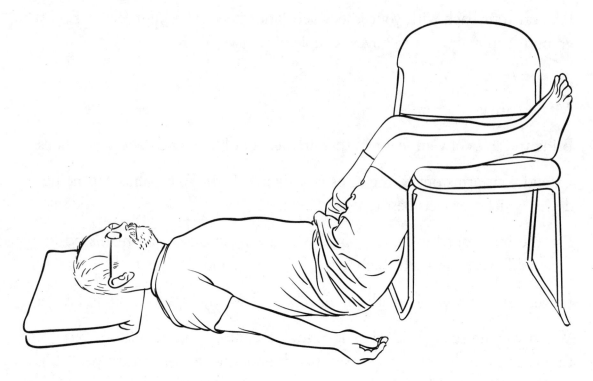

Figure 11.26 Legs on a Chair pose

Setup

Rest on your back with your knees bent, feet flat on the ground, near a stable chair.

Movement

Place your calves on the seat of the chair. Relax your arms at your sides (see figure 11.26).

Breathe.

Spend as much time here as feels comfortable.

When you are ready, hug your knees to your belly.

Place the soles of your feet flat on the ground and roll to one side.

Pause here for a few breaths before coming up to a seated position.

Remember

- If you have long legs, try placing your calves on the chair from the side rather than the front.

- Place a pillow or towel under your head if your chin is jutting up.

Caution

- If lifting your legs onto a chair feels uncomfortable, or if your legs are swollen from a condition such as congestive heart failure, you might try just slightly elevating your legs on a low surface, such as one or two pillows, rather than placing them on a chair. Please check with your physician if you are unsure whether this pose is appropriate for you (see "Partnering with Your Health Care Provider," page 24).

CHAPTER 12

Continuing Your Journey

Now that you have completed six-plus weeks of Relax into Yoga, your practice can become even more interesting as you explore different ways to build your own personalized program. Every day you might choose a different kind of practice to nourish and support yourself, depending on how you are feeling and what is going on in your life. Some days you may feel quite energetic, and a more vigorous practice will serve you best. Other days, you may feel less lively or even fatigued; on these days, you may want a quieter practice that will help you connect with, and gently tend to, your body. Or you may want a practice that includes both quieting postures and a few invigorating poses to enliven your energies. There can also be days when you feel tense or not very grounded. For these days, you may choose a practice that will help you release tension and bring a sense of stability.

To get you started, we have included some suggested sequences drawn from the postures you have been practicing. Once you're familiar with these sequences, feel free to be creative by designing your own practice, considering what serves you best. We encourage you to always start with the Foundational Practice to warm up (Three Part Breath and Range-of-Motion Sequence), then do postures from weeks 2, 3, 4, 5, and 6, then end with Relaxation (page 84). Weeks 2 through 6 can

> Rather than mindlessly moving through life, yoga asks us to be present, pay attention, notice that which is harmful (movements, attitudes, and behaviors) and instead choose that which is supportive.

be considered an à la carte menu: choose what most appeals to you and your body. In this analogy, the Foundational Practice is like the appetizer that stimulates your taste buds in preparation for your meal. The Relaxation pose is the postmeal phase of digesting and integrating the nourishment of your practice. Enjoy.

For your convenience, the instructions and illustrations for the selected poses have been bundled by sequence in individual packets that are available for download at http://www.newharbinger.com/33643.

Rise and Shine

This morning practice is designed to wake up the body and mind and get them ready for the day ahead.

Three-Part Breath (see page 72)

Range-of-Motion Sequence (see page 74)

Supple Spine Flow (see page 148)

Spinal Balance (see page 176)

Mountain (see page 90)

Universal Arms (see page 112)

Side-Angle (see page 98)

Chair Flow (see page 196)

Tree (see page 128)

Crocodile (see page 152)

Baby Cobra (see page 156)

Knees to Chest (see page 162)

Supine Twist (see page 82)

Relaxation (see page 84)

Wind Down

This evening practice is designed to prepare you for deep, restorative rest.

Three-Part Breath (see page 72)

Range-of-Motion Sequence (see page 74)

Supple Spine Flow (see page 148)

Crocodile (see page 152)

Sphinx (see page 154)

Hand to Big Toe (see page 202)

Supine Bound Angle (see page 206)

Supine Twist (see page 82)

Relaxation (see page 84)

Midday Rejuvenation

This is an invigorating practice that will help to enliven your energies.

Three-Part Breath (see page 72)

Range-of-Motion Sequence (see page 74)

Lake Mudra (see page 174)

Knees to Chest (see page 162)

Mountain (see page 90)

Infinity Shoulders (see page 110)

Sun Salutation at the Wall (see page 185)

Crane to Crescent (see page 192)

Tight Rope (see page 142)

Bridge (see page 160)

Knees to Chest (see page 162)

Relaxation (see page 84)

Short and Empowering

Don't let this brief practice deceive you—it can be energizing and very strengthening.

Three-Part Breath (see page 72)

Range-of-Motion Sequence (see page 74)

One-Legged Bicycle (see page 170)

Supple Spine Flow (see page 148)

Plank Progression (see page 180)

Mountain (see page 90)

Warrior 2 (see page 96)

Triangle (see page 100)

Eagle (see page 138)

Baby Cobra (see page 156)

Bridge (see page 160)

Knees to Chest (see page 162)

Relaxation (see page 84)

Short and Sweet

This brief, gentle practice is perfect for times when your body needs extra TLC.

Extended Exploration

When you have the luxury of time, this practice is a very thorough one.

Three-Part Breath (see page 72)

Range-of-Motion Sequence (see page 74)

Supple Spine Flow (see page 148)

Spinal Balance (see page 176)

Plank Progression (see page 180)

Mountain (see page 90)

Salutation Arms (see page 92)

Chair Flow (see page 196)

Warrior 2 (see page 96)

Side-Angle (see page 98)

Triangle (see page 100)

Warrior 3 (see page 134)

Tree (see page 128)

Crocodile (see page 152)

Baby Cobra (see page 156)

Locust (see page 158)

Knees to Chest (see page 162)

Lake Mudra (see page 174)

Hand to Big Toe (see page 202)

Bridge (see page 160)

Knees to Chest (see page 162)

Supine Twist (see page 82)

Relaxation (see page 84)

Afterword

The philosopher George Santayana wrote, "Spirit can enter a human being perhaps better in the quiet of old age and dwell there more undisturbed than in the turmoil of adventure." Santayana's statement reflects the widespread recognition among diverse cultures that as human life advances through age-related phases, the process is accompanied by special growth opportunities. This truth is also highlighted in the ancient yogic texts, which describe "the four stages of life" (*ashramas*). The stages are student, householder, retirement, and renunciation. According to yoga philosophy, retirement is an opportunity for individuals to hand over household responsibilities to the next generation and to gradually transition from a lifestyle focused on income, security, and material pleasure to one that emphasizes a deepening of spiritual practices. Ultimately, as physical abilities decrease with age, individuals ideally enter the stage in which they renounce all other pursuits and devote themselves fully to cultivating spiritual maturity, including profound peace of mind.

Given this ancient yogic perspective, Kimberly and Carol have crafted their Relax into Yoga program for seniors to not only focus on gentle practice of the physical aspects of yoga but also to foster mindful awareness—bringing careful moment-to-moment attention to the full range of experience, including thoughts, emotional currents, the quality of breath, and sensory feedback from one's body.

Based on my immersion in the yoga tradition for twenty years as a swami (monk/teacher), followed by twenty-plus years of work as a clinical psychologist and researcher, I am certain that many aspects of yoga practice are readily accessible for most people, regardless of their cultural background, and also quite effective for helping them feel more ease and joy, and to function better despite chronic illness. Rigorous studies that we have published concur with the findings of other scientists: that yoga practices can improve pain, fatigue, emotional distress, sleep disturbances, and other symptoms among people living with conditions such as metastatic cancer, fibromyalgia, chronic low-back pain, and other illnesses.

As a result of this research, many traditional medical institutions—such as the Oregon Health & Science University, where Kimberly and I work—are rapidly integrating yoga into their programs as a complementary therapy. This book will therefore be very useful not only to yoga teachers and older adult yoga practitioners but also to the growing number of psychologists, social workers, physical therapists, and other professionals who are seeking to weave yoga practices into their offerings.

As this expansion of integrative medicine continues, we will hear more and more accounts of the kind of transformation that occurred for one of my patients. Debbie was a sixty-one-year-old registered nurse who had been forced into retirement by a combination of fibromyalgia and low-back pain. She also suffered from persistent anxiety related to her traumatic childhood. However, as she learned to meditate daily and to work mindfully with her breath throughout the day, she found that her pain began to improve and that she could more easily tolerate the pain that persisted. Debbie's energy level gradually improved, her thoughts were no longer centered on a sense of distress, and ultimately she entered a phase of profound inspiration. She had always had artistic inclinations, but suddenly she found herself producing award-winning sculptures and jewelry. She has now launched a very successful second career and feels very grateful for what she has gained from her yoga practices. As you develop on your yoga journey, my hope is that you too will find rich benefit in your practices and relax into yoga.

—Jim Carson, PhD
Associate Professor, Departments of
Anesthesiology & Perioperative Medicine and Psychiatry
Oregon Health & Science University

Acknowledgments

We are grateful for the wisdom, generosity, and kindness of many wonderful people who contributed to this book. In particular, we offer heartfelt thanks to the visionaries at Duke Integrative Medicine (IM) for their encouragement and support of our efforts to bring the healing benefits of yoga into mainstream medical care. Deep gratitude to Duke IM's founding executive director, Tracy Gaudet, MD; current executive director, Adam Perlman, MD, MPH; program director Linda Smith, PA-C; program coordinator Katie Strobush; chefs Cate Smith and Rebecca Blackwell; business manager Delores Austin; custodian Simon Morko; health center administrator Teresa Keever, RN; and the wonderful Guest Services team for their help in making our Therapeutic Yoga for Seniors Professional Trainings so successful.

Thanks also to the Duke University Medical Center experts who have given so generously of their time and knowledge. For their ongoing support, we are deeply grateful to our core faculty: Mitchell Krucoff, MD; Kathy M. Shipp, PT, MHS, PhD; Francis Keefe, PhD; Jeffrey Browndyke, PhD; Rebecca Crouch, DPT; Rebecca Byrd, DPT; Linda Cates, MS, PT, NCS; Tony Galanos, MD; and Arif Kamal, MD. For their contributions over the years, we would also like to thank Sam Moon, MD, MPH; Anne Kenyon; Evangeline Lausier, MD; Katherine S. Hall, PhD; Kim Huffman, MD, PhD; Gretchen Kimmick, MD; Harold G. Koenig, MD; Matthew Peterson, PhD; Beth Silberman, PT; Burton L. Scott, MD, PhD; Patrick Smith, PhD; Jessica P. Wakefield, MA, LPC; Shelley Wroth, MD; Tara Dickinson, PT, DPT, CCS; Betsy Alden, DMin; Julie Kosey, MS, RYT; and Janet Schaffer, LAc. Our students are among our best teachers, and we offer sincere thanks and warm hugs to those who have shared their yoga journey as panelists during our trainings, including Don Foard, Marilyn

Hartman, Patricia Simmons, Ted Purcell, and Julius "Jack" Raper. Special thanks to Sam Sather, BSN, E-RYT, for her help with managing our certification program.

We are grateful to the Kripalu Center for Yoga and Health for making our training accessible to more yoga teachers. *Namaste* to Rasmani Orth, EdD, and Luke Breslin, as well as Kali Girasek and Sheryl Rapee-Adams. Thanks, too, to Jim and Lynea Gillen of Yoga Calm for sponsoring our abridged training.

For their work in establishing yoga as a respected therapy, we offer admiration and gratitude to the International Association of Yoga Therapists—with special thanks to executive director John Kepner and cofounders Larry Payne, PhD, and Richard Miller, PhD, for encouraging our efforts to make the practice available and appropriate for older adults. Thanks also to the excellent editorial team at New Harbinger, particularly Jess O'Brien, Jess Beebe, Clancy Drake, Jesse Burson, and Vicraj Gill. We are grateful to Marisa Solís for her skillful, meticulous copyediting and to illustrator Lynn Shwadchuck for her lovely drawings. Thanks to our models Jim Carson, Liz Downey, Cynthia Ferebee, Len Ludwig, Mary Jane Ott, Bruce Reavis, Jane Wachsler, and Kathy Williams for their patience, enthusiasm, and generosity in so beautifully illustrating the varied expressions of yoga postures.

Kimberly's Acknowledgments

I extend deep gratitude to the wise and brilliant souls who have nourished me along this journey. Thanks to my Duke colleagues John Barefoot, PhD; Francis Keefe, PhD; and Laura Porter, PhD, for weaving me into the academic behavioral medicine community and encouraging my research passions so wholeheartedly; and to Gwynn Sullivan, RN, MSN, and Jeffrey Brantley, MD, for so graciously welcoming me onto the yoga and mindfulness-based stress reduction teams at the Duke Center for Living. Thank you, Tracy Bogart, for asking me to teach Yoga for Seniors so many years ago and for your inspired and deep knowing that Carol and I "needed to meet." I offer sincere appreciation for my OHSU colleagues Susan Hedlund, MSW, LCSW, OSW-C; Tina Kauffman,

PA, PhD; Carl Davison; Bill Rubine, MS, PT; Kim Jones, RNC, PhD; and Jeffrey Kirsch, MD, for your support, confidence, and friendship. It is a pleasure and an honor to work with you. Thank you to André and Gianna Ripa, for deepening my dance with Spirit. With great love and respect for my primary meditation teachers, I thank Lee Lyon, Mickey Singer, and Joel Morwood; without your clarity and guidance my service in the world would have a very different tone. I bow deeply to the great twentieth-century teachers of the yogic tradition who have illuminated my path: Bhagawan Nityananda, Swami Muktananda, Swami Kripalvananda, and Sri Nisargadatta Maharaj. Thank you to my first teachers, my dear parents, for your love and support along this wild, unpredictable journey. Finally, it is with eternal gratitude that I thank Jim, Grace, and Shankara—the most exquisite and vibrant family I could imagine.

Carol's Acknowledgments

Sincere thanks to Miriam C. Morey, PhD, senior fellow at the Duke Center for Aging and Human Development, and her staff at the Durham VA's Gerofit program, who invited me to become their "Yoga Lady," launching my journey into this transformative endeavor. Warm hugs to gifted nurse-practitioner Suzie Crater, who connected me with the Gerofit team and offers continued inspiration. I'm grateful for the support of extraordinary colleagues at Duke Integrative Medicine and cherish being part of this pioneering group of healers. I offer deep appreciation to the many yoga teachers I've studied with for more than forty years, in particular my mentor Esther Myers, her teacher Vanda Scaravelli, and her teacher T. K. V. Desikachar. Heartfelt gratitude to my late mother, Eleanor Ostrinsky, who was one of my most challenging and best yoga students, for her devotion, courage, and deep love, which are stronger than death. I am grateful for my wonderful son, Max, daughter, Rae, son-in-law, Peter, and dearest Kate, whose light illuminates my world. And eternal thanks to my remarkable husband, Mitchell, for his extraordinary vision, unwavering support, and boundless love.

Resources

How to Find a Well-Qualified Yoga Teacher

Yoga's booming popularity has brought with it a huge surge in classes—some of which are taught by instructors with minimal training in yoga and/or the physiology of aging. To gain the benefits of yoga and minimize the risks, be sure you are working with an experienced, well-qualified instructor in a class that is at an appropriate level for your abilities. Ask prospective teachers how long they've taught yoga, where they studied, if they have experience teaching older adults, and, equally important, how long they've practiced yoga. Authentic yoga instruction is rooted in a teacher's own yoga practice, and the best yoga teachers live their yoga on and off the mat. You might want to observe a class before you participate, and be sure to communicate with the teacher any health considerations that might affect your practice.

Consider trying classes offered at a hospital wellness center or integrative medicine facility. Many offer general yoga classes as well as classes designed specifically for groups, such as cancer survivors, people with heart disease, or those with arthritis. Yoga studios and senior centers often offer classes designed for "mature" bodies, with names like "Yoga Over 50," "Gentle Yoga," or "Senior Yoga."

In addition, try these resources:

Yoga for Seniors is a network of yoga teachers dedicated to making yoga practices available and appropriate for older adults. Founded by Kimberly Carson and Carol Krucoff, the organization's mission is to advance the art and science of adapting the yoga practice to older bodies, minds, and spirits. They offer training programs to help yoga teachers learn how to work safely and effectively with older adults, as well as an intensive certification program for yoga teachers who wish to become Certified Integrative Yoga for Seniors Instructors. For more information, and to locate a graduate in your area, please visit http://www .yoga4seniors.com.

The **International Association of Yoga Therapists** supports research and education in yoga and serves as a professional organization for yoga teachers and yoga therapists worldwide. The organization's mission is to establish yoga as a recognized and respected therapy. To find a yoga therapist in your area, visit its website, http://www.iayt.org.

The **Yoga Alliance** is an organization that registers both individual yoga teachers and yoga teacher-training programs (schools) that have complied with minimum educational standards. For referrals to yoga instructors in your area, visit its website, http://www.yogaalliance.org.

How to Find Trusted Medical Information

The Internet offers a wealth of medical information—some excellent and some completely false. To find reputable information, look for sites sponsored by the federal government (ending in .gov), educational institutions (ending in .edu), or professional organizations (ending in .org). Be cautious of sites with a monetary agenda—that is, those that sell products or services that stand to benefit from information the sites provide.

Here are a few trusted sites:

Medline Plus: The National Institutes of Health's website for patients, their families, and their friends offers information about diseases, conditions, and wellness issues in many languages. You can find out about latest treatments, get information about medications, and view medical videos and illustrations. https://www.nlm.nih.gov/medlineplus.

HealthFinder: This federal government website is managed by the U.S. Department of Health and Human Services and offers resources on a wide range of health topics selected from about 1,400 government and nonprofit organizations. Its mission is "to bring you the best, most reliable health information on the Internet." http://www.healthfinder.gov.

PubMed: A service of the National Library of Medicine and the National Institutes of Health, this site includes more than 25 million citations from MEDLINE and other life science journals for biomedical articles dating back to the 1950s. PubMed includes links to full text articles and other related resources. http://www.ncbi.nlm.nih.gov/pubmed/.

How to Get the Accessories for Your Book

The audio recordings, printable copies of the sequences, Teacher's Guide, and other online materials for this book are available for free at the publisher's website: http://www.newharbinger.com/33643. If you're having trouble using that site, just visit http://www.newharbinger.com/book-accessories for a step-by-step guide to registering your book. Then you can download these helpful materials onto your computer, tablet, and/or smartphone.

References

1. National Center for Complementary and Integrative Medicine. 2008. "Yoga for Health." *NCCIH Publication No. D472*. Updated 2013.

2. ClinicalTrials.gov. n.d. Search results from the U.S. National Institutes of Health. https://www.clinicaltrials.gov/ct2/results?term=yoga&pg=5.

3. Patel, N. K. 2012. "The Effects of Yoga on Physical Functioning and Health-Related Quality of Life in Older Adults: A Systematic Review." *Journal of Alternative and Complementary Medicine* 18: 902–917.

4. Liu, X. C., L. Pan, Q. Hu, W. P. Dong, J. H. Yan, and L. Dong. 2014. "Effects of Yoga Training in Patients with Chronic Obstructive Pulmonary Disease: A Systematic Review and Meta-Analysis." *Journal of Thoracic Disease* 6: 795–802.

5. Medco Health Solutions. 2011. "America's State of Mind." http://apps.who.int/medicine docs/documents/s19032en/s19032en.pdf.

6. Werner, Carrie. 2011. "The Older Population: 2010." *Report No. C2010BR-09*. U.S. Census Bureau.

7. Ortman, J., V. Velkoff, and H. Hogan. 2014. "An Aging Nation: The Older Population in the United States." *Report Number P25–1140*. U.S. Census Bureau.

8. Ibid.

9. Hobbs, F., with B. Damon. 1996. "Current Population Reports: 65+ in the United States." http://www.census.gov/prod/1/pop/p23–190/p23–190.pdf.

10. Clarke, T. C., L. I. Black, B. J. Stussman, P. M. Barnes, and R. L. Nahin. 2015. "Trends in the Use of Complementary Health Approaches Among Adults, United States 2002–2012." *National Health Statistics Reports 79*. Hyattsville, MD: National Center for Health Statistics.

11. National Osteoporosis Foundation. n.d. "Osteoporosis and Your Spine." http://nof.org /articles/18.

12. American Heart Association. 2015. "Protect Your Heart in the Heat." http://www .heart.org/HEARTORG/Conditions/More/MyHeartandStrokeNews/Protect-Your -Heart-in-the-Heat_UCM_423817_Article.jsp.

13. Centers for Disease Control and Prevention and the Merck Company Foundation. 2007. *The State of Aging and Health in America 2007: Executive Summary*. Whitehouse Station, NJ: The Merck Foundation.

14. de Jong, M. R., M. van der Elst, and K. A. Hartholt. 2013. "Drug-Related Falls in Older Patients: Implicated Drugs, Consequences, and Possible Prevention Strategies." *Therapeutic Advances in Drug Safety* 4: 147–154.

15. NIHSeniorHealth. n.d. "Falls and Older Adults." http://nihseniorhealth.gov/falls/about falls/01.html.

16. Broad, William, 2012. "How Yoga Can Wreck Your Body," *New York Times Magazine*, January, 5.

17. Ornish, D., S. E. Brown, J. H. Billings, L. W. Scherwitz, W. T. Armstrong, T. A. Ports, S. M. McLanahan, R. L. Kirkeeide, K. L. Gould, and R. J. Brand. 1990. "Can Lifestyle Changes Reverse Coronary Heart Disease? The Lifestyle Heart Trial." *Lancet* 336: 129–133.

18. American Heart Association. 2015. "About Heart Attacks." http://www.heart.org /HEARTORG/Conditions/HeartAttack/AboutHeartAttacks/About-Heart-Attacks _UCM_002038_Article.jsp.

19. National Cancer Institute. 2014. "Statistics." Division of Cancer Control & Population Sciences, Office of Cancer Survivorship. http://cancercontrol.cancer.gov/ocs/statistics/ statistics.html.

20. National Center for Health Statistics. 2009. *Health, United States, 2008: A Report of the Department of Health and Human Services*. Hyattsville, MD: National Center for Health Statistics.

21. Xu, J. Q., K. D. Kochanek, S. L. Murphy, and E. Arias. 2014. "Mortality in the United States, 2012." *NCHS Data Brief 168*. Hyattsville, MD: National Center for Health Statistics.

22. World Health Organization. 2014. "World Health Statistics 2014." http://www.who.int mediacentre/news/releases/2014/world-health-statistics-2014/en.

23. Arias, E. 2014. "United States Life Tables, 2010." *National Vital Statistics Reports* 63. Hyattsville, MD: National Center for Health Statistics.

24. Krucoff, C., K. Carson, M. Peterson, K. Shipp, and M. Krucoff. 2010. "Teaching Yoga to Seniors: Essential Considerations to Enhance Safety and Reduce Risk in a Uniquely Vulnerable Age Group." *Journal of Alternative and Complementary Medicine* 16: 1–7.

25. Satchidananda, Sri Swami. 2012. *The Yoga Sutras of Patanjali, Translation and Commentary*. Buckingham, VA: Integral Yoga Publications.

26. Mitchell, Stephen. 1991. Tao Te Ching. New York: HarperPerennial, 76.

27. American Heart Association. 2015. "Physical Activity Improves Quality of Life." http://www.heart.org/HEARTORG/GettingHealthy/PhysicalActivity/StartWalking/Physical-activity-improves-quality-of-life_UCM_307977_Article.jsp.

28. Butler, Robert. 2009. Phone interview by Carol Krucoff, June.

29. Butler, Robert. 2010. *The Longevity Prescription*. New York: Avery Books.

30. Mazzeo, R. S. 2007. "Exercise and the Older Adult." *ACSM Current Comment*. Indianapolis, IN: American College of Sports Medicine.

31. NIHSeniorHealth. n.d. "Exercise: Benefits of Exercise." http://nihseniorhealth.gov/exerciseforolderadults/healthbenefits/01.html.

32. Go4Life. n.d. "Do Exercise and Physical Activity Protect the Brain?" National Institute on Aging. https://go4life.nia.nih.gov/tip-sheets/do-exercise-and-physical-activity-protect-brain.

33. Academy of Medical Royal Colleges. 2015. *Exercise: The Miracle Cure and the Role of the Doctor Promoting It*. London: Academy of Medical Royal Colleges, 12. http://www.aomrc.org.uk/doc_download/9821-exercise-the-miracle-cure-feb-2015.html.

34. Holme, I. 2015. "Increases in Physical Activity Is as Important as Quitting Smoking Cessation for Reductions in Mortality in Elderly Men: 12 Years of Follow-Up of the Oslo II Study." *British Journal of Sports Medicine* 49: 743–8.

35. Centers for Disease Control and Prevention. 2015. "FastStats: Exercise or Physical Activity." Early release of selected estimates based on data from the *National Health Interview Survey, 2014*. National Center for Health Statistics. http://www.cdc.gov/nchs/fastats/exercise.htm and http://www.cdc.gov/nchs/data/nhis/earlyrelease/earlyrelease201506_07.pdf.

36. National Center for Health Statistics. 2011. *Health, United States, 2010: With Special Feature on Death and Dying*. Hyattsville, MD: National Center for Health Statistics.

37. Centers for Disease Control and Prevention. 2015. "How Much Physical Activity Do Older Adults Need?" Division of Nutrition, Physical Activity, and Obesity. http://www.cdc.gov/physicalactivity/everyone/guidelines/olderadults.html.

38. Centers for Disease Control and Prevention. 2015. "Physical Activity for Arthritis." http://www.cdc.gov/arthritis/pa_overview.htm.

39. Centers for Disease Control and Prevention. 2012. "Yoga Activity Card." http://www.cdc.gov/bam/activity/cards/yoga.html.

40. Krucoff, C. "Yoga for Seniors Can Help with Balance, Agility, and Strength. But Injuries Do Happen." *Washington Post*, August 18.

41. National Institute on Aging. 2008. "Talking with Your Older Patient: A Clinician's Handbook." *NIH Publication No. 08–7105*. Bethesda, MD: National Institutes of Health, Department of Health and Human Services.

42. U.S. Department of Health and Human Services. 2004. *Bone Health and Osteoporosis: A Report of the Surgeon General.* Rockville, MD: U.S. Department of Health and Human Services, Office of the Surgeon General.

43. National Institutes of Health. 2015. "What Are the Symptoms of a Heart Attack?" National Heart, Lung, and Blood Institute. http://www.nhlbi.nih.gov/health/health-topics/topics/heartattack/signs.

44. Praemer, A., S. Fumer, and D. P. Rice. 1999. *Musculoskeletal Conditions in the United States.* Rosemont, IL: American Academy of Orthopaedic Surgeons.

45. Genant, H. K., C. Cooper, Poor G., I. Reid, G. Ehrlich, J. Kanis, et al. 1999. "Interim Report and Recommendations of the World Health Organization Task-Force for Osteoporosis." *Osteoporosis International* 10: 259–264.

46. National Osteoporosis Foundation. n.d. "Just for Men." http://nof.org/articles/just formen.

47. Penn State Hershey Medical Center. 2013. "Osteoporosis Highlights." http://pennstate hershey.adam.com/content.aspx?productId=10&pid=10&gid=000018.

48. National Osteoporosis Foundation. n.d. "Medicines That May Cause Bone Loss." http://nof.org/articles/6.

49. U.S. Department of Health and Human Services. 2004. *Bone Health and Osteoporosis: A Report of the Surgeon General.* Rockville, MD: U.S. Department of Health and Human Services, Office of the Surgeon General.

50. Ibid.

51. Ibid.

52. National Osteoporosis Foundation. n.d. "Low Bone Density." http://nof.org/articles/9.

53. U.S. Preventive Services Task Force. 2011. "Osteoporosis: Screening." *Annals of Internal Medicine* 154: 356–364.

54. Fechtenbaum, J., C. Cropet, S. Kolta, B. Verdoncq, P. Orcel, and C. Roux. 2005. "Reporting of Vertebral Fractures on Spine X-Rays." *Osteoporosis International* 16: 1823–1826.

55. National Institutes of Health. 2014. "How Does Physical Activity Help Build Healthy Bones?" https://www.nichd.nih.gov/health/topics/bonehealth/conditioninfo/Pages/activity.aspx.

56. Schultz, A. B., G. B. J. Andersson, K. Hadersperk, R. Örtengren, M. Nordin, and R. Björk. 1982. "Analysis and Measurement of Lumbar Trunk Loads in Tasks Involving Bends and Twists." *Journal of Biomechanics* 15: 669–675.

57. Melton, L. J., E. Y. S. Chao, and J. Iane. 1998. "Biomechanical Aspects of Fractures." In *Osteoporosis: Etiology, Diagnosis, and Management*, edited by, B. J. Riggs and L. J. Melton. New York: Raven Press.

58. National Osteoporosis Foundation. 2013. "Moving Safely." In *Bone Basics*. Washington, D.C.: National Osteoporosis Foundation.

59. Centers for Disease Control and Prevention. 2015. "Arthritis-Related Statistics." http://www.cdc.gov/arthritis/data_statistics/arthritis-related-stats.htm.

60. Centers for Disease Control and Prevention. 2015. "Physical Activity for Arthritis." http://www.cdc.gov/arthritis/basics/physical-activity-overview.html.

61. U.S. National Library of Medicine, National Institutes of Health. 2014. "Osteoarthritis." http://www.nlm.nih.gov/medlineplus/osteoarthritis.html.

62. U.S. National Library of Medicine, National Institutes of Health. 2014. "Rheumatoid Arthritis." http://www.nlm.nih.gov/medlineplus/rheumatoidarthritis.html.

63. Ibid.

64. Centers for Disease Control and Prevention. 2015. "Rheumatoid Arthritis (RA)." http://www.cdc.gov/arthritis/basics/rheumatoid.htm.

65. National Institute of Arthritis and Musculoskeletal and Skin Diseases. 2014. "Questions and Answers About Fibromyalgia." *NIH Publication No. 14–5326.*

66. Centers for Disease Control and Prevention. 2015. "Fibromyalgia." http://www.cdc.gov/arthritis/basics/fibromyalgia.htm.

67. National Institute of Arthritis and Musculoskeletal and Skin Diseases. 2014. "Questions and Answers About Fibromyalgia." *NIH Publication No. 14–5326.*

68. Ibid.

69. Carson, J. W., K. M. Carson, K. D. Jones, R. M. Bennett, C. L. Wright, and S. M. Mist. 2010. "A Pilot Randomized Controlled Clinical Trial of the Yoga of Awareness Program in the Management of Fibromyalgia." *Pain* 151: 530–539.

70. Westby, Marie. 2015. "Exercise and Arthritis." American College of Rheumatology. Atlanta, GA: American College of Rheumatology.

71. National Institute of Arthritis and Musculoskeletal and Skin Diseases. 2014. "Joint Replacement Surgery: Health Information Basics for You and Your Family." *NIH Publication No. 14–5149-E.*

72. American Academy of Orthopaedic Surgeons. 2015. "Total Hip Replacement." http://orthoinfo.aaos.org/topic.cfm?topic=a00377.

73. Mayo Clinic. 2014. "First Nationwide Prevalence Study of Hip and Knee Arthroplasty Shows 7.2 Million Americans Living with Implants." http://www.mayoclinic.org/medical-professionals/clinical-updates/orthopedic-surgery/study-hip-knee-arthroplasty-shows-7-2-million-americans-living-with-implants.

74. U.S. National Library of Medicine, National Institutes of Health. 2014. "Taking Care of Your New Hip Joint." https://www.nlm.nih.gov/medlineplus/ency/patientinstructions/000171.htm.

75. Centers for Disease Control and Prevention. 2015. "Chronic Obstructive Pulmonary Disease." http://www.cdc.gov/copd/index.html.

76. American Lung Association. 2013. *Trends in COPD (Chronic Bronchitis and Emphysema): Morbidity and Mortality.* Epidemiology and Statistics Unit Research and Health Education Division. http://www.lung.org/assets/documents/research/copd-trend-report.pdf.

77. Akinbami, L. J., and X. Liu. 2011. "Chronic Obstructive Pulmonary Disease Among Adults Aged 18 and Over in the United States, 1998–2009." *NCHS Data Brief 63.* Hyattsville, MD: National Center for Health Statistics.

78. Centers for Disease Control and Prevention. 2015. "Chronic Obstructive Pulmonary Disease." http://www.cdc.gov/copd/index.html.

79. Paulwels, R. A., and K. Rabe. 2004. "Burden and Clinical Features of Chronic Obstructive Pulmonary Disease (COPD)." *Lancet* 364: 613–620.

80. COPD Foundation. 2015. "Breathing Techniques." http://www.copdfoundation.org/What-is-COPD/Living-with-COPD/Breathing-Techniques.aspx.

81. Bouhassira, D. M. Lantéri-Minet, N. Attala, B. Laurent, and C. Touboulf. 2008. "Prevalence of Chronic Pain with Neuropathic Characteristics in the General Population." *Pain* 136: 380–387.

82. Institute of Medicine. 2011. *Relieving Pain in America: A Blueprint for Transforming Prevention, Care, Education, and Research.* Washington, D.C.: The National Academies Press.

83. U.S. National Library of Medicine. 2015. "Pain Medications: Narcotics." https://www.nlm.nih.gov/medlineplus/ency/article/007489.htm.

84. Keefe, F. J., M. E. Rumble, C. D. Scipio, L. A. Giordano, and L. M. Perri. 2004. "Psychological Aspects of Persistent Pain: Current State of the Science." *Journal of Pain* 5: 195–211.

85. Lumley, M. A., J. L. Cohen, G. S. Borszcz, A. Cano, A. M. Radcliffe, L. S. Porter, H. Schubiner, and F. J. Keefe. 2011. "Pain and Emotion: A Biopsychosocial Review of Recent Research." *Journal of Clinical Psychology* 67: 942–968.

86. Lehrer, P., R. Carr, D. Sargunaraj, and R. L. Woolfolk. 1994. "Stress Management Techniques: Are They All Equivalent, or Do They Have Specific Effects?" *Biofeedback and Self-Regulation* 19: 353–401.

87. Ibid.

88. Gracely, R. H., M. E. Geisser, T. Giesecke, M. A. B. Grant, F. Petzke, D. A. Williams, and D. J. Clauw. 2004. "Pain Catastrophizing and Neural Responses to Pain Among Persons with Fibromyalgia." *Brain* 127: 835–843.

89. Berger, N. A., P. Savvides, S. M. Koroukian, E. F. Kahana, G. T. Deïmling, J. H. Rose, K. F. Bowman, and R. H. Miller. 2006. "Cancer in the Elderly." *Transactions of the American Clinical and Climatological Association* 117: 147.

90. American Cancer Society. 2014. *Cancer Treatment & Survivorship Facts & Figures*. Atlanta, GA: American Cancer Society.

91. Busch, V., W. Magerl, U. Kern, J. Haas, G. Hajak, and P. Eichhammer. 2012. "The Effect of Deep and Slow Breathing on Pain Perception, Autonomic Activity, and Mood Processing: An Experimental Study." *Pain Medicine* 13: 215–228.

92. Martin, S. L., K. L. Kerr, E. J. Bartley, B. L. Kuhn, S. Palit, E. L. Terry, J. L. DelVentura, and J. L. Rhudy. 2012. "Respiration-Induced Hypoanalgesia: Exploration of Potential Mechanisms." *Journal of Pain* 13: 755–763.

93. Zautra, A. J., R. Fasmana, M. C. Davisa, and A. D. Craig. 2010. "The Effects of Slow Breathing on Affective Responses to Pain Stimuli: An Experimental Study." *Pain* 149: 12–18.

94. Lumley, M. A., J. L. Cohen, G. S. Borszcz, A. Cano, A. M. Radcliffe, L. S. Porter, H. Schubiner, and F. J. Keefe. 2011. "Pain and Emotion: A Biopsychosocial Review of Recent Research." *Journal of Clinical Psychology* 67: 942–968.

95. Lehrer, P., R. Carr, D. Sargunaraj, and R. L. Woolfolk. 1994. "Stress Management Techniques: Are They All Equivalent, or Do They Have Specific Effects?" *Biofeedback and Self-Regulation* 19: 353–401.

96. Raghavendra, R. M., R. Nagarathn, H. R. Nagendra, K. S. Gopinath, B. S. Srinath, B. D. Ravi, S. Patil, B. S. Ramesh, and R. Nalini. 2007. "Effects of an Integrated Yoga Programme on Chemotherapy-Induced Nausea and Emesis in Breast Cancer Patients." *European Journal of Cancer Care* 16: 462–474.

97. Carson, J. W., K. M. Carson, L. S. Porter, F. J. Keefe, H. Shaw, and J. M. Miller. 2007. "Yoga for Women with Metastatic Breast Cancer: Results from a Pilot Study." *Journal of Pain & Symptom Management* 33: 331–341.

98. Carlson, L. E., and S. N. Garland. 2005. "Impact of Mindfulness-Based Stress Reduction (MBSR) on Sleep, Mood, Stress and Fatigue Symptoms in Cancer Outpatients." *International Journal of Behavioral Medicine* 12: 278–85.

99. Smith, J. E., J. Richardson, C. Hoffman, and K. Pilkington. 2005. "Mindfulness-Based Stress Reduction as Supportive Therapy in Cancer Care: Systematic Review." *Journal of Advanced Nursing* 52: 315–327.

100. Holzel, B. K., S. W. Lazar, T. Gard, Z. Schuman-Olivier, D. R. Vago, and U. Ott. 2011. "How Does Mindfulness Meditation Work? Proposing Mechanisms of Action from a Conceptual and Neural Perspective." *Perspectives on Psychological Science* 6: 537.

101. Davidson, R. J., J. Kabat-Zinn, J. Schumacher, M. Rosenkranz, D. Muller, S. F. Santorelli, F. Urbanowski, A. Harrington, K. Bonus, and J. F. Sheridan. 2003. "Alterations in Brain and Immune Function Produced by Mindfulness Meditation." *Psychosomatic Medicine* 65: 564–570.

102. Grant, J. A., J. Courtemanche, and P. Rainville. 2011. "A Non-Elaborative Mental Stance and Decoupling of Executive and Pain-Related Cortices Predicts Low Pain Sensitivity in Zen Meditators." *Pain* 152: 150–156.

103. Holzel, B. K., U. Ott, T. Gard, H. Hempel, M. Weygandt, K. Morgen, and D. Vaitl. 2008. "Investigation of Mindfulness Meditation Practitioners with Voxel-Based Morphometry." *Social Cognitive & Affective Neuroscience* 3: 55–61.

104. Holzel, B. K., U. Ott, H. Hempel, A. Hackl, K. Wolf, R. Stark, and D. Vaitl. 2007. "Differential Engagement of Anterior Cingulate and Adjacent Medial Frontal Cortex in Adept Meditators and Non-Meditators." *Neuroscience Letters* 421: 16–21.

105. Buckwalter, J. A. 1995. "Aging and Degeneration of the Human Intervertebral Disc." *Spine* 20: 1,307–1,314.

106. Twomey, L. T., and J. R. Taylor. 1987. "Age Changes in Lumbar Vertebrae and Intervertebral Discs." *Clinical Orthopaedics and Related Research* November: 97–104.

107. Nair, S., M. Sagar, J. Sollers III, N. Consedine, and E. Broadbent. 2014. "Do Slumped and Upright Postures Affect Stress Responses? A Randomized Trial." *Health Psychology* 34: 632–641.

108. Percia, M., S. Davis, and G. Dwyer. 2012. "Getting a Professional Fitness Assessment." *ACSM Fit Society* Spring edition. American College of Sports Medicine.

109. NIHSeniorHealth. n.d. "Falls and Older Adults." http://nihseniorhealth.gov/falls/about falls/01.html.

110. National Institute of Arthritis and Musculoskeletal and Skin Diseases. 2015. "Handout on Health: Back Pain." *NIH Publication No. 15–5282.* Bethesda, MD: National Institutes of Health.

About Our Relax into Yoga Models

Jim Carson, PhD, sixty-four, is a clinical psychologist and a former swami (monk) in the yoga tradition. He weaves the practice of meditation into his work in helping individuals cope with chronic medical illnesses such as cancer, fibromyalgia, and low-back pain. He has published several studies documenting the positive impact of yoga and meditation on persistent pain, fatigue, and emotional distress. Jim says, "The deep joy and peace that arises in my daily practice continues to be the bedrock of my life."

Lillian "Liz" Downey, seventy-one, is a retired financial-aid administrator and adjunct lecturer. She has been a yoga student in the senior yoga class at the Durham Center for Senior Life for several years, and she says that the practice of yoga has helped relieve a knee problem and also has been an ongoing form of exercise for good health. She is inspired by deep meditation and overall well-being of body and mind.

Cynthia Ferebee, sixty-eight, began studying and practicing yoga in 2009 after retiring from teaching in the public school system for more than thirty-five years. She now teaches beginning yoga at the Durham Center for Senior Life. Yoga has helped Cynthia manage and decrease the pain associated with arthritis and other common ailments that come with aging. Cynthia is dedicated to helping other seniors acquire and maintain greater flexibility and peace of mind through a consistent yoga practice that includes meditation, breathing exercises, and body posturing.

Len Ludwig, seventy-eight, is a semiretired owner/executive of an equipment financing company. His engineering and finance background trained him to think very logically, and he says he has "been constantly amazed at the whole new world opened up to me, starting about one year ago, with a class about mindfulness." As a result of practicing what he has learned in this new dimension, he reports improvements in his breathing, relaxation, flexibility, and general well-being. He looks forward to learning more.

Mary Jane Ott, seventy, retired after fifty years in the field of nursing, forty of which she worked and taught as a nurse practitioner in a variety of clinical settings. She continues to consult as an integrative nurse coach and to offer yoga and meditation classes. Mary Jane enjoys a full and active life with family and friends as she pursues creative, intellectual, and spiritual interests. Living with health challenges from traumatic injuries, she is grateful for her many years of yoga and meditation practices, which continue to be a foundational part of her daily self-care, maximizing her health, spiritual, and functional abilities.

Bruce E. Reavis, sixty-eight, was involved in a severe motorcycle accident after retiring as a career counselor for the state of North Carolina and as a fitness coordinator. He sustained several broken bones in his leg, arm, shoulder, and pelvis that required multiple operations. Along with prescribed physical therapy, Bruce included yoga in his regimen. Just when his dedication to yoga began to give him greater flexibility, he was diagnosed with stage IV lymphoma. It did not devastate him. He continued his yoga practice through the chemo treatments, and the lymphoma has been in remission since 2013. Although he is living with cardiac issues, he attributes his ability to maintain a positive outlook to his yoga experience and his belief in a gracious God.

Jane Wachsler, seventy-eight, was born in the Midwest, graduated with a teaching degree from the University of Michigan–Ann Arbor, and spent the next few years teaching children with special needs. After raising her three daughters, she worked for the Metropolitan Museum of Art in a program that served the needs of children and adults with multiple disabilities. She left the museum after thirty-three years to care for her husband, who had Parkinson's disease, and they moved from the East Coast to the West Coast to be with their grandchildren. After her husband died, Jane was diagnosed with breast cancer; she has recovered well and is traveling as much as possible.

Kathy Williams, fifty-nine, is a retired teacher/counselor who worked in the Durham, North Carolina, public schools. After retirement, she made a commitment to "live." One part of that commitment is to practice yoga daily both on and off the mat. She has found that practicing yoga every day has helped her live a holistic and healthy lifestyle. She is more relaxed, breathes slower, has increased energy, sleeps better, eats healthier, and has better balance and flexibility. Since Kathy started practicing yoga, her sinus problems have decreased tremendously. And, "More important," she says, "yoga has helped me have peace of mind." Meditation has enabled her to see things differently, with positive feelings and attitudes.

Kimberly Carson, MPH, E-RYT, is a health educator at Oregon Health & Science University (OHSU) in Portland, OR, specializing in the therapeutic use of yoga and mindfulness meditation for seniors and people with medical challenges. She currently offers classes to cardiac, oncology, and chronic pain patients. Kimberly has developed and taught yoga programs being researched at Duke University Medical Center and OHSU. The *Yoga of Awareness* program, developed by Kimberly and her husband Jim, has been shown in research trials to significantly reduce pain and fatigue in women with metastatic breast cancer, breast cancer survivors, as well as women with fibromyalgia. For more information, please visit her website at www.mindfulyogaworks.com.

Carol Krucoff, E-RYT, is a yoga teacher at Duke Integrative Medicine in Durham, NC, where she specializes in therapeutic applications of yoga for people with health challenges. An award-winning health journalist, Carol served as founding editor of *The Washington Post*'s Health Section, and her articles have appeared in numerous national publications, including *The New York Times*, *Yoga Journal*, and *Reader's Digest*. She is author of several books, including *Yoga Sparks* and *Healing Yoga for Neck and Shoulder Pain*, and is creator of the audio home-practice CD, *Healing Moves Yoga*. For more information, please visit her website at www.healingmoves.com.

Kimberly and Carol are codirectors of *Yoga for Seniors*, a network of yoga teachers dedicated to making yoga practices appropriate and available for older adults. They are codirectors of *Integrative Yoga for Seniors Professional Training*, and cocreators of the DVD, *Relax into Yoga for Seniors*. For more information, please visit their website at www.yoga4seniors.com.

Foreword writer **Mitchell W. Krucoff, MD**, is professor of medicine/cardiology at Duke University Medical Center, and codirector of the Cardiovascular Devices Group at Duke Clinical Research Institute. He is internationally recognized for his pioneering research in computer-assisted heart monitoring, new modalities of coronary revascularization, and cardiovascular applications of spiritual and complementary therapies. Author of more than 250 publications in the cardiology literature and book chapters in medical texts, Mitchell is senior editor of the *Journal of Alternative and Complementary Medicine*. He has served on the board of directors of the Sri Sathya Sai Institute of Higher Medical Sciences in Puttaparthi, India, since its construction in 1990, and is a fellow of the American College of Cardiology, the American Heart Association, and The Society of Coronary Angiography and Interventions. Mitchell is a special government employee of the United States Food and Drug Administration, from whom he received a Distinguished Award for his tenure on the Circulatory Devices Advisory Panel. He has been married to Carol Krucoff since 1974, and they have two adult children.

Afterword writer **Jim Carson, PhD**, is a longtime student of Swami Muktananda. He is a former yogic monk who has taught the practices and philosophy of yoga worldwide for over thirty years. Now a clinical health psychologist and associate professor of anesthesiology at Oregon Health & Science University (OHSU), Jim is applying his expertise to the development and evaluation of yoga and meditation-based clinical treatments. He has worked extensively with patients suffering from persistent pain, including those with cancer, fibromyalgia, and multiple sclerosis. While Jim was on faculty at Duke University, he and his wife Kimberly developed the *Yoga of Awareness* program, and completed research trials with metastatic breast cancer patients and survivors of early-stage breast cancer. During his tenure at OHSU, a successful research trial has been completed using *Yoga of Awareness* for fibromyalgia. Jim and Kimberly together developed the first mindfulness program for couples, as well as the first loving-kindness meditation program for medical patients.

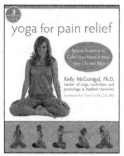
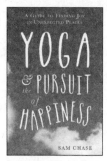
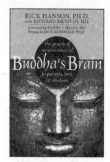
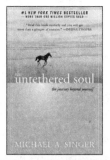
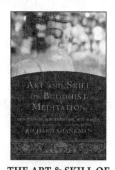
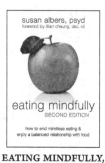

Register your **new harbinger** titles for additional benefits!

When you register your **new harbinger** title—purchased in any format, from any source—you get access to benefits like the following:

- Downloadable accessories like printable worksheets and extra content

- Instructional videos and audio files

- Information about updates, corrections, and new editions

Not every title has accessories, but we're adding new material all the time.

Access free accessories in 3 easy steps:

1. Sign in at NewHarbinger.com (or **register** to create an account).

2. Click on **register a book**. Search for your title and click the **register** button when it appears.

3. Click on the **book cover or title** to go to its details page. Click on **accessories** to view and access files.

That's all there is to it!

If you need help, visit:

NewHarbinger.com/accessories

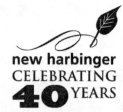

new harbinger
CELEBRATING
40 YEARS